The Ethos of Medicine in Postmodern America

Philosophical, Cultural, and Social Considerations

Arnold R. Eiser

LEXINGTON BOOKS
Lanham • Boulder • New York • Toronto • Plymouth, UK

Published by Lexington Books
A wholly owned subsidiary of Rowman & Littlefield
4501 Forbes Boulevard, Suite 200, Lanham, Maryland 20706
www.rowman.com

10 Thornbury Road, Plymouth PL6 7PP, United Kingdom

British Library Cataloguing in Publication Information Available

Library of Congress Cataloging-in-Publication Data
Eiser, Arnold R., 1947- author.
The ethos of medicine in postmodern America : philosophical, cultural, and social considerations /
Arnold R. Eiser.
p. cm.
Includes bibliographical references and index.
ISBN 978-0-7391-8180-5 (cloth : alk. paper) -- ISBN 978-0-7391-8181-2 (electronic) I. Title.
[DNLM: 1. Delivery of Health Care--United States. 2. History, 21st Century--United States. 3.
Medical Informatics--United States. 4. Physician's Role--United States. 5. Physician-Patient Rela-
tions--United States. W 84 AA1]
RA418.3.U6
362.10973--dc23
2013037328
ISBN 978-1-4985-2097-3 (pbk : alk. paper)

Printed in the United States of America

Contents

Introduction

The Ethos of Medicine in Postmodern America

What is the Ethos of Medicine in twenty-first century postmodern America? What are the essential operative values in healthcare today? Has postmodern American culture so altered the landscape of medical care that moral confusion and low morale among clinicians have increased faster than technological advancements and ethical resolutions? This book is an attempt to answer these questions and provide some solutions with reference to the cultural touchstones of our postmodern era: consumerism, computerization, the power and influence of corporations with regard to medical practice, and the leveling of the medical hierarchy. Any professional practice is thoroughly embedded in the social and cultural matrix of its society, and the medical profession is no exception. Corporatization, consumerism, and computerization constitute the three C's of postmodern healthcare in the twenty-first century, and their impact needs to be examined both philosophically and sociologically.

I derive many of my observations from the cultural insights of leading postmodern thinkers including Foucault, Lyotard, Baudrillard, Bauman, Levinas, Borgmann, and Jameson. By applying their more general insights to the culture of healthcare delivery, one can get a better understanding of what has transpired in healthcare in the postmodern era. Among postmodern thinkers, only Foucault actually focused his critique on medical care itself and then he did so in the remote past. However the combined analyses of these and other contemporary thinkers provide a valuable perspective for gaining understanding of contemporary changes in healthcare delivery. It is often difficult to fully comprehend what is happening in one's psychosocial-cultural epoch as you experience it directly. Therefore it is useful to have a mediating process for refracting those observations through the lens of another system of thought. I am suggesting here that the prism of postmodern thought offers such a heuristic with which to "view the eclipse" of changing medical practice.

In making this examination, I draw upon of the insights of key Continental thinkers as well as American scholars. I examine a variety of contemporary healthcare issues with regard to how postmodern culture and its critical impacts have changed healthcare attitudes and conduct. While I focus on the changes in America in particular, postmodern changes are occurring on a global scale. Hence I reference studies done in Asia, Australia, Europe, and Africa as well as in the USA and Canada. I do not necessarily endorse the views of postmodernism, but believe much can be learned from the insights of both its proponents and its critics in examining the challenges of healthcare in the 21st century. The cultural milieu in which medicine is practiced has changed very substantially and much can be learned from the perspectives of these cultural interpreters and social philosophers. Furthermore my comments are informed by empirical information from both health services research and the sociology of medicine. I attempt to develop a new understanding of healthcare delivery in the twenty-first century, and suggest some developments that I consider *post-postmodern* that might be nurtured in order to avoid a barren *Silicon Cage* of corporate, bureaucratized medical practice.

My perspectives on healthcare matters are also refracted through the lenses of bioethics, health services research, and healthcare policy as well as through selected experiences that I have had as a clinician, medical educator, clinical researcher, health services researcher, and physician leader. Having long held an interdisciplinary perspective, I hope to bring such a perspective to this discussion of current healthcare issues such as the Patient Centered Medical Home, the Accountable Care Organization, clinical practice guidelines, and electronic health records.

In addition to identifying areas of concern, I provide some suggestions that help preserve the ethos of humane medical practice in this era of postmodern relativism, corporate capitalism, and radical consumerism. The loss of notions of community, altruism, and heroism has lessened the myth of the physician, and challenged the ethical basis of medical practice as employed in the nineteenth and early- and middle-twentieth centuries. Can a new basis for ethical medical practice be initiated that gives voice to patient activation and recognizes the significant role of nurses? The widespread role of computer technology , the focus on consumerism as a deep cultural value, the egalitarian flattening of the hierarchy in clinical medicine, and the burgeoning twenty-first century healthcare corporate bureaucracy are the focal topics of this book.

The shibboleth in healthcare management today is "patient-centered" medical care. It mimics the management dictum of customer focus in other consumer-based industries. Medical sociology as well as bioethics have noted that medical practice in the past was too physician-focused.[1] Sociologists, bioethicists, and a panoply of healthcare corporations have succeeded in derailing physician hegemony, while consumerist ideology has readily advanced an avowed patient focus, if only superficially. However, few patients feel like they are at the center, which suggests that medical care in postmodern America has at its core a business focus, and that "patient-centered" is something of a marketing ploy. The consumer model of healthcare readily fits into the highly consumerist orientation that postmodern society has in general. Individuals express their identity through the objects they own as well as the services they purchase. Baudrillard[2] notes that in postmodern culture one becomes what one buys and that one's selection of possessions distinguishes the individual from others in society whether it is smart phones, computers, designer labels, etc; so it goes with healthcare services, as well where each delivery system aspires to its signature services.

The consumerist model is a poor substitute for a thicker notion of the patient-physician relationship based on community values, altruism, authority derived from self-sacrifice, and high standards of professionalism. It is not realistic to recommend a return to the values and culture of the nineteenth and twentieth centuries. Rather, one can and should explore what can be done in the twenty-first century to reconstruct a sound basis for medical practice in a humane and compassionate manner, and how the practice of medicine, retaining a primary essence of professionalism, can incorporate an emphasis on greater teamwork. Is it possible in this era of for-profit corporate medicine, electronic health records, online ratings and blogs, and multiple stakeholders? Exploring the culture of medicine as well as societal cultural change at large will help illuminate the limits of what can or should be done to renew the ethos of medical practice in the twenty-first century.

A "meta-awareness" of the cultural impact of societal changes on clinical processes is the key to finding innovative solutions. There is a need to address the issue of how a pluralistic society develops a thicker notion of the common good than is currently possible, or at least develop a *modus operandi* that permits some ethical agreement in the public sphere of clinical practice. The exponential growth of the medical-industrial complex is simply not sustainable within our economy, and we have reached those limits sooner than many imagined. How can our postmodern culture, imbued with moral relativism, be coaxed toward some thicker consensus of the common good that restrains the exponential growth of medical costs? Exploring key issues affecting the culture of medicine and their social matrix may provide the basis for a renewed ethos of medical practice in the twenty-first century.

The loss of grand narratives (Lyotard) and the awareness of power inequalities and their implications and tenacity (Foucault) have added to the difficulty of building a consensus of opinion. Some of the differences are

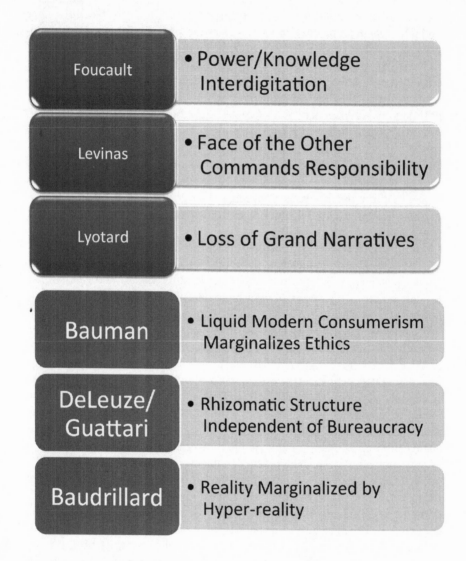

Figure 0.1. Postmodern Thinkers

inter-generational rather than strictly based on political alignment. A shift in attitudes away from a singular professional focus toward work-life balance has occurred with a majority of members of the millennial generation under contemporary social influences, which certainly includes the computerized exchange of digital information and images e.g. Facebook and its psychological impact as well as those of multiculturalism, corporate capitalism, and loss of community.

Postmodernism has been long on critique and short on recommendations to correct the shortcomings of our current circumstances. By contrast, my approach is syncretic, consequentialist, and pragmatic. I make some positivist recommendations that include, among others, a combination of appreciative inquiry and adaptive leadership, mindfulness techniques in medicine, transparency in the roles and responsibilities of patients as well as providers, and approaches that help reduce the negative impact of the mechanistic, technocratic, computerized bureaucracy (the Silicon Cage) as well as focusing on Levinas's call to acknowledge the primacy of responsibility for the Other.

In this century of accelerated change, advancing computer technology, and exponential information expansion, there is a need to develop a new understanding of the ethos of medicine. This is an exploration worth undertaking, and one that, I believe, will invoke some fresh approaches to critical issues in delivering medical care in the twenty-first century and the possibilities and challenges that it evokes.

ACKNOWLEDGMENTS

I thank my wonderful wife, Barbara J. A. Eiser, for copyediting this work. I also thank my friends who offered helpful suggestions and encouragement: William Fuentevilla, JD; Edward Huth, MD, MACP; Jeffrey Brensilver, MD, FACP; and Michael Parmer, MD, FACS. Arthur Caplan, PhD; Jonathan Moreno, PhD; Renee Fox, PhD; and Nora Jones, PhD, offered helpful advice.

I extend my thanks to Jana Hodges-Kluck, editor for Lexington Books at Rowman & Littlefield, and Jay Song, assistant editor, for seeing the merit in this work and their efforts in bringing it to press. Anonymous reviewers provided useful comments that I gratefully acknowledge, too.

I also note that I could not have written this book without postmodern computer technology. While I critique computer technology, data analysis, and bureaucracy, I recognize their value when experienced in moderation with wisdom and restraint.

NOTES

1. Katz J. *Silent World of Doctor and Patient*. Johns Hopkins U. 2002.
2. Baudrillard J. "Consumer Society," in Selected Writings. M. Poster, ed. (Cambridge: Polity Press, 1988) 29.

Chapter One

The Ethos of Medical Practice in the Age of Computerized Technology

"Modern technology has become a total phenomenon for civilization, the defining force of a new social order in which efficiency is no longer an option but a necessity imposed on all human activity." —Jacques Ellul[1]

"Power is not an institution, and not a structure; neither is it a certain strength we are endowed with; it is the name that one attributes to a complex strategic situation in a particular society." —Michel Foucault[2]

BACKGROUND

Computerization of the medical record has developed fitfully in the highly segmented, competitive marketplace in the United States healthcare "system." While a nationally uniform electronic health record (EHR) has been implemented for many years in a number of Western European countries, the widespread usage of EHRs has not been the same in the USA.[3] In the USA computerization has been caught in the "vortex of the money economy" rather than being a part of a carefully considered national health policy. Commercially marketed computer systems have proliferated in this burgeoning and profitable industry. Creswell notes that the profitability of the EHR vendors follows successful lobbying efforts for the usage of EHRs to require a federal mandate for computerization.[4] This culminated when the Center for Medicare and Medicaid Services (CMS) issued a series of bonus payments and payment penalties rules regarding the usage of EHRs in 2011, and meaningful computerized medical information use became required in 2012 in order to foster adoption of EHRs[5] by both physician practices and hospitals. Healthcare organizations have proceeded to acquire EHRs with Computer-

1

ized Physician Order Entry (CPOE) with Clinical Decision Support Systems (CDSS) at considerable cost for both the purchase and implementation of these complex computer systems.[6] Computerized order entry is the part of the EHR wherein the physician or mid-level provider orders medications, fluids, imaging studies, laboratory tests, and other clinical procedures. CDSS is a component computer program that uses some form of artificial intelligence to integrate medical knowledge into some control over what items are ordered for a patient. A metanalysis of CDSS studies revealed that a majority of published reports (68 percent) showed positive results in improving processes of care.[7] Of course publication bias, which favors the publication of positive results may have influenced this finding. Currently it is estimated that an EHR system has a life expectancy of six years so that computerization will undoubtedly raise the cost of healthcare before it begins, if ever, to lower it.

Bureaucracies, both public and private, are growing in size and authority concordant with the growth of information technology. The rationale behind using CPOE with CDSS is that a knowledgeable committee of informed experts can craft an order set for the patient with specific disorders that would be better than a set of orders crafted by individual physicians. This reflects the prevailing faith in expert panels crafting clinical practice guidelines based on the latest evidence-based medical studies. A few obstacles present themselves to such an approach. First, when patients are admitted to the hospital, diagnoses on the first day are rarely certain yet the order sets need to placed then before all the pertinent clinical and laboratory results are back. As opposed to individualized orders written by independent medical professionals who may "hedge" their orders in a manner that addresses more than one diagnosis, a standardized order set will have more rigidity than "free text" ordering thus limiting such a syncretic approach. Boyd et al. pointed out that problems arise when patients with multiple disorders have clinicians attempting to follow several guidelines simultaneously. Conflicting guidelines may negatively impact such patients particularly when they are elderly and otherwise more susceptible to adverse effects of medications and other components of treatment guidelines.[8] Researchers in the field have also noted such unintended consequences as new types of entry errors, lack of previous cross checks by the nurse, overdependence on technology, and changes in the power structure.[9]

The clinicians, the healthcare system clinical information executives, and the vendors of complex EHR systems all have differing objectives as they approach the enormous technological changes in healthcare delivery. Clinicians must contend with the clinical and human needs of the patient as well as with their own remuneration and professional status, while the corporate executives are concerned on the return on investment (ROI) of expensive computer systems, and the EHR vendors are concerned with sales and profits. A crucial question must be considered as a result of these factors: has the corporate computerization of medical practice compromised medical professionalism?

If physicians in pursuit of the compliance with CPOE with DCSS do not sufficiently vary their treatment approach to account for individual fragility and variability, then patients may not benefit from such an approach to care. The question at hand is whether an established computerized, corporately authorized order set inhibits clinical professionalism to some extent. It is reasonable to ask: at what stage of medical computerization does a clinician capable of professional judgment and responsibility transform into a technocrat?

David Blumenthal, CEO of the Commonwealth Fund and the former National Coordinator of Health Information Technology in the Obama administration, has noted that the information technology revolution of the past two decades has reduced the mystique of the physician and could reduce the patient's trust in the clinician.[10] So if information technology such as the Internet is de-mystifying medical knowledge for patients, at least to some extent, how does that impact the professional status of clinicians? For one thing it is likely to disproportionately affect primary care physicians (PCPs) although specialists are also affected. The knowledge/power equation differential for primary care physicians is different because of the breadth of medical issues that may present to PCPs. In addition, the lack of specialization limits the depth of their knowledge in any one subject except for the most common conditions in their practice such as hypertension and diabetes management. In contrast, specialists generally possess certain procedural skills within their domain that are essential to certain diagnostic and therapeutic interventions. As a result, the power differential between specialist and generalist may become enhanced in an era of widespread information technology.

For ambulatory clinicians, the odds are more likely that their computerized information systems will not be connected to a hospital's EHR or to that of the specialists they consult unless they practice within a large integrated healthcare system. Although primary care physicians are now acquiring EHRs at a record pace, it is an expensive acquisition and the return on the investment for them is uncertain. It is another deterrent to the independent practice of primary care in the twenty-first century and the increasing role for medical corporations to become the predominant mode of clinical practice. Healthcare systems are acquiring primary care practices and some specialty practices at a record pace as well. Whether this will produce better clinical care remains to be determined, but it will undoubtedly change the essence of clinical practice and the affective quality of clinical care. Physicians will increasingly become employees of healthcare systems rather than independent practitioners. Some may hail such as an improvement but beware of unexpected consequences including lower levels of patient connectedness and engagement.

INFORMATION TECHNOLOGY IMPLICATIONS

Information technology itself can have hidden challenges as well as the more apparent benefits. Baudrillard, the French social theorist and critic of technology and consumerism, noted the danger of computer technology's penchant for simulation. He calls attention to the postmodern consumer's devotion to simulations of reality, termed hyperreality.[11] Is there a risk that the increased computerization of medical information, medical records, and order sets will create a clinical simulacra that eclipses the actual patient? Could a physician driven by the rules of CPOE, CMSS, and P4P create a "patient simulacra" that becomes a totem of her/his attention to a greater extent than the actual patient? Boyd et al.'s[12] simulation suggests it could be a real concern. Baudrillard noted that there is an intoxicating quality to hyperreality that can alter the sensibilities and perceptions of those captured by the virtual imagery of the technological creation.[13] Could this happen as the computerization of clinical care advances in the next decade? I am reminded of a recent occasion when a medical school lecturer arrived a few minutes later and the students would not let her stop the videotape of her lecture from a previous year for her live talk. Have we indeed already developed a penchant for electronic versions of reality?

Perhaps one should check some of the unbridled enthusiasm for computerized medicine as it creates the perfect environment for increased bureaucratic control of medical practice and the potential erosion of the professionalism of medicine. Our fascination with the computerized information technology can have unanticipated effects that are both operational and psychological in nature. The crisis in medical care in the United States is not only financial in nature. It includes challenges to the power and knowledge of clinicians as well as how they interact with a computerized nexus of clinical information and how this alters the interpersonal and professional nature of clinical practice. Computerized order entry using predetermined order sets alters the power equation in favor of the healthcare bureaucracy and a complicated web of for-profit and government bureaucracies that deliver, fund, assess, and measure healthcare activities. Increasingly, medical orders are no longer the product of an independent professional's judgment and responsibility, but are determined by a nexus of power corporate relationships and are therefore socially and politically constructed. Grant notes that computer technology "harnesses language for quantitative evaluation"[14] so that it is no longer subjected to qualitative values such as justice, freedom, or virtue. McLuhan's admonition that the medium is the message rings as true today as it did fifty years ago.[15] Finally, as Calhoun notes, citing Foucault, all knowledge is an exercise of power[16] and medical informatics is hardly an exception. It may be the best example of this phenomenon yet in medicine or anywhere in our social milieu.

CLINICAL OUTCOMES AND ELECTRONIC HEALTH RECORDS

Consider the state of the evidence that health information technology improves medical care processes and clinical outcomes. A systematic review of the subject by Chaudry et al. notes that much of the positive results in health information technology come from four benchmark institutions who developed their own computer infrastructure.[17] In contrast, studies of commercially available EHR products were less likely to have produced statistically valid positive outcomes data with these products. Some well-done studies of this type produced results that did not show improvement with the computerized approach.[18,19] One study even showed that new types of errors can occur with CPOE including double dosing orders and inflexible ordering format leading to medication errors.[20] It has been commonly known for some time that it is easier to write an order for the wrong patient with CPOE since there is no physical chart to pick up per se and one can easily click on the drug or dosage next to the one intended. Of note also is that the articles referenced in the Chaudry metanalysis on this subject had little information regarding the cost to computerize medical records and orders. It will undoubtedly cost in the billions of dollars nationally and will be a recurring cost as well. One can only speculate why there is such a paucity of such cost information in these studies but the power/knowledge equation is no doubt not far away from the answer.

A recent systematic review notes that despite the impressive number of health information system studies, "the cumulative evidence on the quality of care continues to be mixed and contradictory."[21] Regarding clinical outcomes in their analysis, sixty-four percent of the studies revealed no positive effects of the EHR on morbidity or mortality, eighty-two percent showed no positive effect on psychological or physiological measures, and 100 percent showed no improvement in the quality of patients' lives. Provider productivity was more likely to be reduced as it takes longer to make discrete computerized entries. Discrete entry is necessary for the data to be manipulated. Moreover, the overall quality of the information content was just as likely to be reduced as improved and it was often necessary to add "free-text" to fully capture accurately the clinical picture.

It is fair to ask whether the narrative of computerization of medical ordering and medical records has not become the major postmodern cultural myth. This has occurred despite the claims of postmodernism that overarching narratives are finished. Apparently when it comes to consuming computer technology, mythology is alive and robust. The hero of the myth has merely transformed from the physician to the computer technology. Postmodern sensibility includes the presupposition that technology and computerization are always superior.

Thus, medical information is under an imperative to be digitized in the twenty-first century. Jameson has described postmodernism as the "cultural logic of late capitalism."[22] Late capitalism is multi-national, media savvy, computer technology-dependent, and market-oriented. Ideology and science merge in the postmodern capitalist colonization of other spheres of life including science, technology, think tanks, universities, entertainment/news information businesses, architecture, healthcare, and almost everything else through the vehicles of consumerism and capitalization. Do not the assumptions concerning EHR benefits reflect the cultural hegemony of computerization? Is this not connected to corporate advocacy and profiting from computerized commercial processes?

For those who find this line of analysis too Marxian, consider a more traditional capitalist approach. Adam Smith identified three virtues underlying happiness: justice (fair and equitable), beneficence, and prudence (avoiding unnecessary risk and exercising self-control).[23] The Invisible Hand of traditional capitalism contained these virtues. If they are sufficiently lacking then capitalism, according to Smith, is likely to run amok.[24] Postmodernist business perspectives are more concerned with profitability, marketability, and computerization than justice, beneficence, and prudence. So classic mercantile capitalism also views current global capitalism with concern.

Have we exercised self-control, justice, beneficence, and avoidance of unnecessary risk in the coercive marketing of the EHR? In line with Foucault, Armstrong observes: "Power assumes a relationship based on some knowledge which creates and sustains it; conversely power establishes a particular regime of truth in which certain knowledges become admissible or possible."[25] The "regime of truth" in our times heavily favors computerization, demanding a type of knowledge to accompany consumption of software programs in healthcare, and clinicians will follow this path whether they find it helpful or not.

There is a dark side to vigorously pursuing the proliferation of computerized medical records.

Consider the following:

- Computerization enables the storage of a very large amount of data that can be obtained systematically by a "hacker" or computer intruder.
- Remote access of such information is made possible by network computer systems.
- Much of the information is of a private nature.[26]

- The leaking of private patient information is commonplace and reported regularly in the media.

In Massachusetts, over one million people have had medical records, credit cards, and other personal information revealed by Blue Cross/Blue Shield of Massachusetts as well as by banks.[27] New York Presbyterian Hospital/Columbia University Medical Center had a security lapse that allowed personal information belonging to as many as 6,800 former patients to be published on the Internet.[28] These are but a few of the many instances that have occurred. No hospital or healthcare system, or for that matter any organization that deals with digitized information, is immune to such leaks even though there are laws and procedures to provide security against them. The technology makes the information accessible in ways that a paper chart could never do.

COMPUTERIZATION AND BUREAUCRACY

Computerization of medical records is part of a much larger process, viz. the bureaucratization of healthcare delivery that has been in progress for more than two decades. Max Weber, the seminal sociologist of organizations and bureaucracies, observed that documents and files are central to the operation of a bureaucracy.[29] Bureaucracy thrives on information gathering, centralization of control, and implementation of standardized protocols, and computerization makes all of that eminently more possible and almost instantaneous. Weber, while perceiving benefits of bureaucracies, also noted they tended toward power aggrandizement with resultant power plays, and were prone toward degeneration into oligarchy where rational rules yield to administrative fiat. Frederick, a scholar of managerial values and business ethics, refined the notion of power aggrandizement[30] noting that it is both a strength and a weakness of the modern corporation. He noted that it is pro-entropic promoting the accrual of power at the expense of the maximization of production. Its strength relates to the "chieftain" power to control those under his/her authority. He speculates that it owes that strength to a genetic tendency to respond to male assertiveness, although several females have mastered the craftsmanship of corporate leadership and assertiveness in the postmodern era.

Undoubtedly, the computerization of medical records will continue to accelerate the bureaucratization of medical care to an as yet unprecedented degree. It is no mere coincidence that the patient safety/quality improvement movement did not take off until computers were in full scale use for the past two decades even though Ernest Codman first suggested an approach to improving patient safety more than a century ago.[31] Dr. Codman was the Boston surgeon who first suggested the assessment and transparent reporting of surgical outcomes in 1906, raising the ire of both his fellow surgeons and the hospital board. For his efforts, that includes starting the first Morbidity and Mortality Conference where outcomes of surgical cases were reviewed as a departmental activity, Dr. Codman lost his hospital privileges from the Massachusetts General Hospital. Thereafter quality improvement initiatives laid dormant for much of the century.[32] Codman is also credited with helping start the American College of Surgeons as well as the forerunner to the Joint Commission and he made several other notable contributions to practice improvement. Certainly he challenged the authority and autonomy of the surgeons and the hospital in an era when that was not considered appropriate by societal standards. In every era there is a cost for challenging authority, but progress does not occur unless someone has the courage to do so.

Consider, if you will, a contemporary analysis of healthcare bureaucracy. An analysis by Kitchner, Caronna, and Shortell describes a typology of the modes of physician control in healthcare systems.[33] First in temporal order is the mode of custodial control characterized by a high degree of physician autonomy, quality assessment by physicians, fee for service practice, and low use of clinical software. The bureaucracy in this mode is subservient to the physician professionals. Contrasted with this is what the authors term the "heterogeneous" mode characterized by little physician autonomy, managerial systems with benchmarking, quality assessment of physicians by managers using computer software, and the use of industrial methods of total quality management. Healthcare systems in the past decade have clearly gravitated toward the heterogeneous mode with the use of software programs such as Crimson Physician Software analytics,[34] using the techniques of statistical quality control to assess individual physicians at system hospitals and outpatient centers. These authors, as well as Light and Levine,[35] note that the bureaucratization of medical care was abetted by physicians' pursuit of income growth as well as the countervailing forces from the growth of the managed care industry including both health maintenance organizations (HMOs) and preferred provider organizations (PPOs). Certainly computer usage was vital to the growth of the concept and implementation of "managed care" as well as the quality improvement movement. Technology today, as always, has a major role in shaping social values and societal practices. One can expect both benefits and problems from the implementation of a technological, computerized approach to healthcare delivery. Only time will tell wherein rests the balance.

ROLE OF BIOETHICS

Alongside the role of computers and insurance companies in the de-professionalization of physicians, the illuminating disclosures of bioethics have contributed to the distrust of physicians. Books such as *The Silent World of Doctor and Patient*[36] by Jay Katz MD, JD decried the paternalism and arrogance of the medical profession and *Strangers at the Bedside: A History of How Law and Bioethics Transformed Medical Decision Making*[37] by David Rothman documented how the rise of patients' rights were woven into the fabric of the American legal system in view of the rise of bioethics and consumer rights. These insights and the ensuing policy changes were certainly a necessary corrective to the excesses of physician paternalism. Nevertheless this development added another element to the reduction of the diminishing moral voice of the physician. The transformation of the physician role may have been inevitable as the growth of the technology of medicine required huge capital investment that individual practioners would not be able to meet. Thus, macro- and micro-economics as well as social, bioethical, and legal forces combined to rewrite the role of the physician as an important technocrat in a system of healthcare rather than as an independent professional. Computerization has had a large role in this and will continue to expand over the next generation through not only EHRs but several other software applications that expand the role of the bureaucracy, expanding its authority and reach into clinical care, with both positive and negative effects. The fact that centralization of decision-making rarely has an entirely salutary effect on organizations has already been shown.[38]

An insight into the two polarities of American ethos can be found in Alasdair McIntyre's *After Virtue*.[39] He notes that there are two modes of social life in contemporary culture: "one in which the free and arbitrary choices are sovereign" (read: patient autonomy in the medical realm) and the "one in which the bureaucracy is sovereign, precisely so that it may limit the anarchy of self-interest" (read: insurance company requirements for prior authorization of medical procedures). So with the physician reduced to the role of the technocrat, American medical care oscillates between the autonomous choice of lifestyle (obesity, riding motorcycles without helmets, substance abuse, risky sex, demands for futile medical care near the end of life) and bureaucratic control by insurance plans attempting to maximize profits and reduce their costs and liabilities. Nevertheless these influences come together to maintain the medical-industrial complex as well as the growth of clinical and academic medicine both with their business interests and connections. McIntyre noted that with the end of communal life in America, and the predominance of law and bureaucracy, the era of social learning of virtue is now past and prudential judgment in social life is in rare supply.[40] This combination of willful entropic freedom combined with market-based solutions contributes to the exponential growth of healthcare in America. Lack of restraint in healthcare consumption is a necessary consequence of combining autonomous lifestyles choices, bureaucratic for-profit control of healthcare delivery, and diminished moral voice in the postmodern era.

PERSONAL PERSPECTIVES, LEGAL ASPECTS, AND
TECHNOCRATIC MANAGERALISM

Personal perspectives also influence the response to computerization. Dent noted that the implementation of the same computer technology in two different renal units was experienced with differing degrees of acceptance by the physicians and nurses depending on the specific characteristics of the groups of nurses and the groups of physicians.[41] The physicians in one group who were oriented toward research and education embraced the technology, and the nurses in the other group who favored quality assessment embraced the information technology while the physicians in the latter group were hostile. So individual characteristics of healthcare providers rather than just the type of provider, physician, or nurse, will influence the degree to which the technology is enthusiastically utilized or not. The enthusiasm of clinicians for computerized medical practices then differs substantially among providers of the same type. Computerization may favor both clinical research and quality assessment efforts even if it does not necessarily improve quality but provides more accessible data for analysis.

There are unintended consequences of computerization that one can only begin to comprehend. A recent *New England Journal of Medicine* article[42] mentions the new risks of medical liability associated with the use of electronic medical records. The authors indicate liability risks vary with the stage of implementation. In early stages problems arise with the paper-electronic interfaces, inadequate training, inaccurate inputs, and system malfunctions. As the systems mature, problems arise from the "cutting and pasting" function that perpetuates mistakes, from the more extensive documentation providing more clinical information for discovery, poorly developed mechanisms for e-mail communication with patients, and clinicians adversely affected by information overload and experiencing alert fatigue. As both EHRs and Health Information Networks (HIN) become widespread heightened standards for clinical decision support using established guidelines, and obtaining information from other sources and other computers may not be consistently met. As cases are always individualized by the patient's clinical circumstances, it may prove difficult to "shoehorn" the patient into the computerized order set.

This concern is shared by authors who note that evidence-based medicine advocates have been ideologically driven in downplaying the subjective and individualized aspects of clinical care.[43] These authors speak of a "methodological fundamentalism" and suggest a tangled web between evidence-based medicine (EBM), Pharma, government groups, and lobbies as well as a willing academia and their research sponsors. Denzin, Lincoln, and Giardina[44] raise concern that social science inquiry becomes the "handmaiden of a technocratic, globalizing manageralism." Don't fully computerized medical records lead further in the direction of a technocratic, managerial approach to healthcare replacing the medical professionalism model of the twentieth century? Some may say that is for the best. But one needs to be cognizant of its disadvantages as well, before leaping into the technological, bureaucratic eclipse of the individual professional model of care. Again the insights of Foucault are informative: How much of the knowledge that has been elucidated in randomized clinical trials has been linked to the power influences of the research sponsor? No one author can be entirely certain of the extent. There are skillful ways of "gaming" a large prospective clinical trial especially when one's career depends upon a successful outcome.

Foucault warns us that power and knowledge are inextricably enmeshed in one another. A technology as intrusive as electronic medical information is certainly bound to have its own effect on the power/knowledge equation. It is truly hard to imagine it has no effect. The Health Information Technology for Economic and Clinical Health Act of 2009[45] provides the legal and financial impetus for widespread implementations of EHRs. The widespread change will inevitably "follow the money" and significantly impact clinical practice. Borgman[46] notes that "while information technology is alleviating overt misery, it is aggravating a hidden sort of suffering that follows from the slow obliteration of human substance. It is the misery of persons who lose their wellbeing . . . when moral gravity and the material density of things is overlaid by the lightness of information technology." The insights of these thinkers shed considerable light on the recent developments in healthcare.

Dean commenting on Hardt and Negri's *Empire* notes that in "communicative capitalism the use value of a message is less than its exchange value, its contribution to a large pool, flow or circulation of content. A contribution need not be understood; it need be only repeated, reproduced, and forwarded."[47] This sounds eerily reminiscent of some of the concerns raised regarding the EHR and CPOE and Pay for Performance and their electronic downloads. The communicative flow of medical knowledge is envisioned to improve care and it may do so in selected instances but given humanity's track record for "gaming the system," any system, is well-known; some applications may have less congenial aspects than originally intended.

I am not suggesting that EHRs, computerized order sets, and Health Information Exchanges are not going to be of some value in improving health outcomes. However respected investigators have done careful studies and failed to find significant improvements or cost savings from EHR implementation. DesRoches et al. at Massachusetts General Hospital and the Harvard School of Public Health analyzing the Hospital Quality Alliance database and related databases found very little or no improvement in clinical outcomes whether a hospital had an advanced EHR, basic EHR, or no EHR.[48] Himmelstein and associates found similarly negative results.[49] What I wish to call attention to are two observations: first is that these changes in process will also materially change the roles, attitudes, and values of the clinicians that are integral to healthcare delivery. One cannot change the delivery system in this fashion without also significantly altering how the professionals working in healthcare will think about themselves and how others will view them as well. In fact those changes are already underway. We need to guard against reification of computerization of medical information and give this development as much careful, objective scrutiny as possible. Second, the decision to implement EHRs has occurred in the USA without a careful examination of the data before it was mandated. Its appeal is intuitively obvious but what we have learned in the EBM era is the "intuitively obvious" is not synonymous with true. While we have developed skepticism of physicians and awareness of their fallibility, we have not developed an analogous skepticism of the value of computerization; even so, it has become such an integral part of our professional lives and has subconsciously gained a special status in our postmodern cultural values.

Also we must be vigilant that individuals high on the socioeconomic scale do not benefit more excessively than those lower on the scale. The latter groups should not miss out on benefits or bear an excessive amount of the disadvantages of the computerized health record (This is discussed in more detail in chapter 4). Certainly confidentiality must be safeguarded to a great extent for all patients and that itself will be a greater challenge when medical records are fully digitized. Who can guarantee such safeguards of confidentiality? Certainly laws on this matter may help, but it will also call for resources by healthcare systems that will have many competing demands generated by patient demands, regulatory government demands, and insurance companies' demands for additional data downloads that require increasingly sophisticated information systems and the corresponding technical support. Those lower on the socioeconomic scale could have increased vulnerability as this system evolves.

SUMMARY

In addition to some of the unique features of information technology, I have noted that computerized technology changes both the nature of the patient-physician interaction as well as how both the physician and patient view the professional roles of clinicians. The computerization of medical information fits well Jameson's description of the cultural invasiveness of late capitalism and its "colonization" of other spheres of human life through the power vehicle of consumerism.

Computerization "feeds" the bureaucracy with the growth of clinical and outcomes data and related information. The data so far has not shown that all

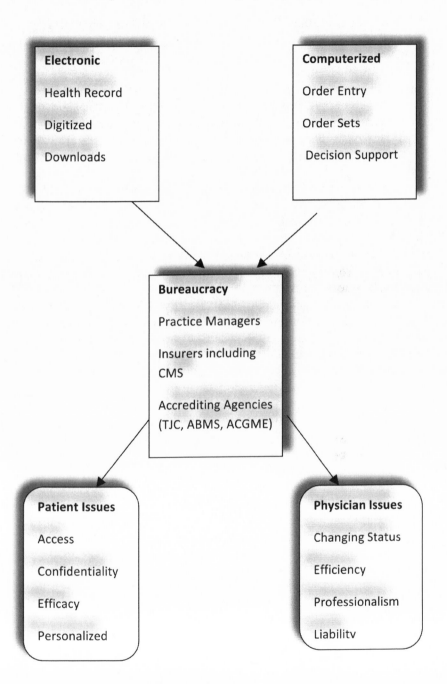

Figure 1.1.   Computerized Medical Practice

these additional data downloads actually improve clinical care outcomes although they may improve processes.

Bioethics was already changing the professional status of the medical profession by challenging its tendency toward paternalism and helping to implement legal changes that assure patients the autonomous rights of consumers. These bioethical and legal changes have acted synergistically with the computerization of healthcare delivery in impacting physician roles and stature. Perhaps it is time for bioethicists to consider the ethical impact of the computerization of medical practice and the growth of centralized bureaucracies.

Computerization of the medical record will have many intended and unintended consequences. Some can be anticipated now and there is a need to discuss them fully and candidly while new effects will be discovered with further implementation. To what extent is computerization of medical information the "handmaiden of a technocratic manageralism"? That is an important question that we need to ponder as a self-reflective society, so we are fully aware of what is developing.

Computerization's impact on clinical care will include changes to the patient/physician relationship, the roles of physicians, and their interactions with multiple stakeholders in the clinical arena, especially patients but also insurers, regulators, healthcare systems, and other parties. Concerns about the confidentiality of digitized data will persist and present new challenges that new laws alone will not necessarily control. The impetus to the changing role of the physician from an independent professional to a sophisticated technocrat will have significant effect on the ethical nature of medical practice. It is difficult to have the final word on this development as it is still an evolving phenomenon but it is one that warrants serious and careful attention.

Moreover, as will be further discussed in another chapter, the need to individualize care for individuals with multiple morbidities requires that physicians retain the ability and the authority to make those modifications to the patient's orders that the standardized computer order sets do not contain. [50]

Another matter to consider is how computerized medical information alters medical education; this will be considered in detail in another chapter. Medical students themselves have noted that the use of computerized order sets discourages thinking about the individual component of orders for patients. [51] It is hard to imagine that such a loss of reflection concerning the components of medical care is going to improve a future physician's understanding of the clinical process. Excessive reliance on computerized ordering threatens to deprofessionalize at least some aspects of being a medical professional.

NOTES

1. Ellul J. *The Technological Society*. New York: Knopf. 1964.

2. Foucault M. *The History of Sexuality. Vol 1. An Introduction*. Trans R. Hurley. London: Penguin, 1980, 90–92. http://www.brainyquote.com/quotes/quotes/m/michelfouc165444.html.

3. Schoen C, Osborn R, Huynh PT, Doty M, Peugh J, Zapert K. On the front lines of primary care: primary care doctors' office systems, experiences, and views in seven countries. *Health Aff* (Millwood) 2006; 25: 555–w57.

4. Creswell J. A digital shift on health data swells profits in an industry. *New York Times*. http://www.nytimes.com/2013/02/20/business/a-digital-shift-on-health-data-swells-profits. html?emc=eta1&_r=0. Accessed March 17, 2013.

5. http://www.healthit.gov/policy-researchers-implementers/meaningful-use Accessed November 4, 2012.

6. Hillestad R., Bigelow J., Bower A., et al. Can electronic medical record systems transform health care? Potential health benefits, savings, and costs. *Health Aff* 24(5):1103–1117, 2005.

7. Hunt D. L., Haynes R. B., Hanna S.E. Effects of computer-based clinical decision support systems on physician performance and patient outcomes. *JAMA* 280(15): 1339–46, 1998.

8. Boyd C. M., Darer J., Boult C., et al. Clinical practice guidelines and the quality of care for older patients with multiple comorbid diseases: Implications for pay for performance. *JAMA* 294: 716–724, 2005.

9. Campbell E. M., Sittig D. F., Ash J. S., Guappone K. P., Dykstra R. H. Types of unintended consequences related to computerized provider order entry. *J Am Med Inform Assoc* Sep–Oct; 13(5): 547–56, 2006.

10. Blumenthal D. Quart doctors in a wired world: Can professionalism survive connectivity? *Milbank Quarterly* 80(3): 525–545, 2002.

11. Jean Baudrillard. "Simulacra and Simulations," in *Selected Writings*, Mark Poster, ed. Stanford: Stanford University Press, 1988, 166–184.

12. Boyd ibid.

13. Baudrillard J. *Simulacra and Simulation,* Ann Arbor: Univ of Mich Press, 1994.

14. Grant I. H. Postmodernism and science and technology, in *Postmodernism*, ed. Stuart Sim. Oxford and New York: Routledge, 2001, 66.

15. McLuhan M. *Medium Is the Message*. London: Penguin, 1967.

16. C. Calhoun. Culture, history, and the problem of specificity in social theory. In *Postmodernism & Social Theory*, Seidman S., Wagner D. G., eds. Oxford: Blackwell, 1992.

17. Chaudry B., Wang J., Wu S., et al. Systemic review: Impact of health information technology on quality, efficiency, and costs of medical care. *Ann Intern. Med 144L* 742–752, 2006.

18. Rollman B. L., Hanusa B. H., Gilbert T. et al. The electronic medical record. A randomized trial of its impact on primary care physicians; initial management of major depression (corrected) *Arch Int Med* 161: 189–197, 2001.

19. Kilgore M. L., Flint D., Pearce R. The varying impact of two clinical information systems in a cardiovascular intensive care unit. *J Cardiovasc. Manag.* 9: 31–5, 1998.

20. Koppel R., Metlay J. P., Cohen A., et al. Role of computerized physician order entry systems in facilitating medication errors. *JAMA* 2005; 293: 1197–1203, 2005.

21. Lau F., Kuziemsky C., Price M., Gardner J. A review of systematic review of health information system studies. *J Am Med Inform Assoc* 17: 637–645, 2010.

22. Jameson F. *Postmodernism, or the Cultural Logic of Late Capitalism.* Durham NC: Duke Univ Press, 1991.

23. Smith A. *Theory of Moral Sentiments:* Indianapolis: Liberty Fund, 1982.

24. Busch M. Adam Smith and Consumerism's Role in Happiness: Modern Society Reexamined. *Major Themes in Economics*. Spring 2007. http://business,uni.edu/Themes/Busch.pdf. Accessed June 2012.

25. Armstrong D. *Bodies of knowledge/knowledge of bodies*, in *Reassessing Foucalt*. C. Jones, R. Porter, eds. London: Routledge, 1994.

26. Protecting the Privacy for Computerized Health Information. US Congress Office of Technological Assessment. 1993. http://www.mccurley.org/papers/9342.PDF accessed November 28, 2010.

27. Bray H. Data breaches affect a million state residents. http://www.boston.com/business/technology/articles/2010/01/03/data_breaches_affect_m.

28. City Apologizes for Information Leak. Asscociated Press. http://newyork.cbslocal.com/2010/09/27/city-hospital-apologizes-for-patients-info-leak/.

29. Weber M. *The Theory of Social and Economic Organization*. Translated by A.M. Henderson and Talcott Parsons. London: Collier Macmillan Publishers, 1947.

30. Frederick W. C. *Values, Nature and Culture in the American Corporation*. New York: Oxford U Press, 1995 p71.

31. Codman E. *A Study in Hospital Efficiency*. Boston, Mass.: Privately printed, 1916.

32. Mallon, B. *Ernest Amory Codman: The End Result of a Life in Medicine*. Philadelphia: WB Saunders, 2000. http://en.wikipedia.org/wiki/International_Standard_Book_Number.

33. Kitchner M., Caronna C. A., Shortell S. M. From the doctor's workshop to the iron cage? Evolving modes of physician control in US health systems. *Soc Scien Med* 60: 1311–1322, 2005.

34. http://www.crimsonservices.com/products.html. Accessed December 1, 2010.

35. Light D., Levine S. 1988. The changing character of the medical profession: A theoretical overview. *The Milbank Quarterly* 66 (suppl. 2): 10–32.

36. Katz J. *The Silent World of Doctor and Patient*. Baltimore: Johns Hopkins Univ Press, 2002.

37. . Rothman D. *Strangers at the Bedside: A History of How Law and Bioethics Transformed Medical Decision Making*. New York: Basic Books, 1991.

38. Zabojnik J. Centralized and decentralized decision making in organizations. *J. Labor Econ.* 20(1): 1–14, 2002.

39. McIntyre A. *After Virtue: A Study in Moral Theory*. South Bend, IN: Notre Dame U Press 1984, 35, 195.

40. Ibid 169–170.

41. Dent M. Organization and change in renal work: A study of the impact of a computer system within two hospitals. *Sociology Health Illness* 12(4): 413–431, 1990.

42. Mangalmurti S. S., Murtagh L., Mello M. M. Medical malpractice liability in the age of electronic health records. *N Engl J Med* 363: 2060–2067, 2010.

43. Murray S. J., Holmes D., Perron A., Rail G. No exit? Intellectual integrity under the regime of 'evidence' and a 'best practices.' *J Eval Clin Pract*. 13: 512–516, 2007.

44. Denzin N. K., Lincoln Y. S., Giardina M. D. Disciplining qualitative research. *Int J Qual Studies in Education* 19(6): 769–782, 2006.

45. Health Information Technology for Economic and Clinical Act of 2009. (HITECH Act) Pub. L No 111-5, Div A Tit XIII,DivB tit IV, Feb 17,2009,123 Stat 226.467 (codified in sections of 42 USCA.

46. Borgmann A. *Holding on to Reality: The Nature of Information at the Turn of the Millennium*. Chicago: Univ Chicago Press, 232, 1999.

47. Passavant P. A., Dean J. eds. *Empire's New Clothes: Reading Hardt and Negri*. New York: Routledge, 274, 2004.

48. DesRoches C. M., Campbell E. G., Vogeli C., et al. Electronic health records' limited successes suggest more targeted uses. *Health Affairs* 29(4): 639–646, 2010.

49. Himmelstein D. U., Wright A., Woolhandler S. Hospital computing and the costs and quality of care: A national study. *Am J Med*. 123(1): 40–46, 2010.

50. Larrriviere D. G., Bernat J. L. Threats to physician autonomy in a performance-based reimbursement system. *Neurology* 70:2338–2342, 2008.

51. Knight A. M., Kravet S. J., Harper G. M., Leff B. The effect of computerized provider order entry on medical student clerkship experiences. *J Am Med Inform Assoc*. 12: 554–560, 2005.

Chapter Two

On the Nature of Medical Knowledge

Evidence-Based Medicine in Postmodern America

"Renewing human society cannot happen in this technologically complex society without the very adult awareness that *someone's* designs will be adopted, that *someone* will make decisions about allocation of resources, and about what lines of research to pursue and which to ignore." —J. M. Staudenmaier[1]

Medical knowledge is not science per se, although it makes use of the biological sciences in deriving clinical practices and designing basic medical research. However, human beings are subject to both the laws of nature and the laws of humankind, both explicit and tacit. The social construction of medical knowledge and clinical practice is a complex multi-factorial, often fractious process that involves many stakeholders. These stakeholders, including physicians, patients, research funders, and policy experts, can conflate medical knowledge including evidence-based medicine with biological science. One noticeable difference between the two is that evidence-based medicine can change dramatically with one or two new well-conducted randomized prospective clinical trials published in a respected journal. Within a year organizations that establish practice guidelines incorporate that new information into the guideline. Science, with few exceptions, changes more slowly and somewhat more decisively.

Foucault accords a pre-eminent role to medicine as the foundation of the social and biological sciences.[2] There may be little historical truth in that, but it is true that in post-revolutionary France the clinical-pathologic "clinical gaze" was born in the wake of the destruction of the "Old Guard" of medical experts. The French public hospital provided the setting for the discovery of the nature of human disease by examining large populations of seriously ill people, recording the clinical descriptions of diseased conditions, combining that with autopsies of the deceased, and describing the accompanying under-lying pathology. Thus clinical medicine was born in that revolutionary time. It was augmented with development of laboratory science from Germany and sterile technique from Scotland.[3] Foucault, in his *Birth of the Clinic,* de-scribes the creation of an apprenticeship model where the teacher merely needed a "certificate of integrity and good citizenship from his municipal-ity."[4] In the hospital, as opposed to the university of the Ancien Regime, philosophy could be removed from medicine and replaced with empirical observation and treatment. As new rules were taking form they required a new syntax and language. Again Foucault notes the uniqueness of the study of medicine:

> It is understandable then, that medicine should have such importance in the constitution of the sciences of man—an importance that is not only methodo-logical but ontological, in that it concerns man's being as an object of positive knowledge. The possibility for the individual of being both the subject and object of his own knowledge implies an inversion in the structure of finitude.[5]

Thus a new way of conceiving, diagnosing, and treating diseases of man was also changing the way humankind conceived of itself as free from central authority except for that found in medical and related sciences. But Foucault also noted that medicine became an instrument of power and control by the administrative bureaucracy, and physicians became agents to some extent of that controlling bureaucracy.[6] Both then and now, if the physician desired access to the patients and facilities of the hospital, he was required to concur with its bureaucratic rules.

This formulation is incomplete, however, unless we return to one of Fou-cault's central theses, that of the interconnectedness of power and knowl-edge.

> Knowledge derives not from some subject of knowledge, but from the power relations that invest it. Knowledge does not "reflect" power relations; it is not a distorted expression of them; it is immanent in them. . . . Power and knowl-edge directly imply one another.[7]

I differ somewhat from Foucault on this point, inasmuch to recognize that power may, in fact, distort knowledge or bias the objectivity of the "clinical gaze" to some extent. I will elaborate on that subsequently.

Foucault's discursive analysis included the "enunciative modality," in that a statement of information is dependent on the *status* of the speaker, the *location* from which the statement emanates, as well as the *position* of the statement in regard to other such statements.[8] Foucault made these comments relating to medicine as well as other subjects. Maseide notes that discursive and collaborative processing of evidence in medical problem solving involves certain fluidity between the rigidly defined scientific guidelines and the practical and ethical aspects of an individual patient's problems.[9] The master clinician may have some tacit knowledge that evades a committee-approved guideline obtained by doing a more thorough subgroup analysis or by considering qualitative elements as well as quantitative ones. Different patients in different life circumstances may influence appropriate clinical choices. Moreover, the patient may be in a subset whose outcomes differ significantly from the population studied in the clinical trial. This is admittedly nuanced and assuredly every clinician is not a master clinician even as we would hope that all are. While healthcare executives would like to eliminate the variances in medical care, human variability as well as the complexity of patients and their illnesses confound such a bureaucratic effort.

Polanyi speaks of ineffable knowledge exemplified by an experienced surgeon who knows the terrain of the body where he has repeatedly operated.[10] Tacit knowledge also exists in other domains of medical expertise. The judgment of the master clinician often is based upon subliminal knowledge of clinical subsets that may pose significant variation from the conventional wisdom underlying a guideline. The guideline may have subtly excluded the individual with her particular set of clinical or personal characteristics. In addition, Polanyi refers to the interpersonal knowledge of two or more people and a component of experience that propositional knowledge cannot capture.[11] Reinders extends this thought to include current quality measurements which discourage the personalized component of clinical care.[12] He goes on to state, along with Friedson,[13] that insisting solely upon objectified quality standards is a form of "organized social distrust" of professionals. So in the milieu of social distrust are we about to exclude important subtypes of medical knowledge?

Davidoff, former editor of the *Annals of Internal Medicine,* addresses the reality of the heterogeneity of clinical medicine which differs from the artificial constraints of randomized clinical trials.[14] He also posits that the discipline of improving health is a social discipline because the care process is the sum of actions by many human agents. He suggests that, to improve clinical practice, what is needed is a "hybrid science" including comparative effectiveness research, Bayesian analysis (a type of statistical inference that makes modifications when additional information becomes available), and pragmatic trials. Pragmatic trials differ from prospective randomized clinical trials by comparing two interventions in everyday clinical settings using a large sample size where not all variables are controlled.[15]

I concur with Davidoff's suggestions and would also add elements of management science to the equation. In fact, even master clinicians are slow to absorb and apply some aspects of evidence-based medicine because of both cognitive and interpersonal reasons, not to mention forms of unconscious bias.

Practice based evidence research methodology (PBRM) is a prospective, observational cohort study that does not seek to limit types of patients or interventions[16] which differs considerably from a randomized clinical trial (RCT). The PBRM creates a heterogeneous data set that more closely resembles clinical practice and then uses multivariant statistical analyses to "clean" the data to make tentative conclusions. Since not every topic in medicine can and will be subjected to an RCT for both economic and practical reasons, this newer methodology is important. Pragmatic clinical trials comprise a type of PBRM that reduces confounders but does not control study variables to the same extent as RCTs. They have the advantage that they are closer to community practice settings[17] and can better address such matters as patient adherence in a general clinical setting. RCTs are assuredly still very much needed but will not answer all clinical questions as many clinical questions are not amenable to this methodology. The federally chartered Patient Centered Outcomes Research Institute (PCORI) recognizes the need for pragmatic trials as well as RCTs.[18]

Investigators have noted problems exist with the manner in which randomized clinical trials are conducted and interpreted. Hayward, Kent, and colleagues have called attention to the need to risk stratify the population studied prospectively and to refine conclusions of efficacy by defined risk profile-based subgroup analysis.[19] If this is not done, both the benefits and the risks for specific patient subgroups may be seriously misinterpreted. Why is this type of analysis not done more often? Some of the reasons include the possibility of various stakeholders having differing motivations, and a degree of inertia toward changing the status quo. In fact, this technique of prospective risk stratification is not commonly performed. Medical science is practiced in the imperfect world of social differences, power inequalities, and plain bad habit but also influenced by the profit motive.

Another challenge to the accuracy of clinical guidelines is that genetic and even racial differences may alter responses to drug therapy.[20] Clinical trials do not usually take this into consideration; even if they do, they are less likely to enroll ethnic groups as subjects. As a result, data concerning such genetic differences are not likely to become apparent during randomized controlled clinical trials where the emphasis is on the randomness of patient selection. So a clinical guideline may be less applicable to a patient in a particular ethnic group that did not participate in the clinical trial cited in the practice guideline. Yet when a RCT becomes part of a broad clinical practice guideline, ignoring genuine ethnic differences may become "imperialistic" and medically inappropriate.

Editors of medical journals possess their own biases that relate to the socio-political environments where they find themselves. For example, when

I wrote an article describing the association of over-expression of TGF-beta growth factor and resultant fibrosis accounting for much of the excessive morbidity and mortality among African Americans,[21] not a single American editor would send it out for review. Why not, you may ask? The American "politically correct" value assumption that African Americans are not genetically different from Caucasians prevented any editor from even considering sending the manuscript out for review, regardless of its scientific merit. In contrast, it was reviewed by all three European journals to which I sent it, including *The Lancet,* where two reviewers called it important, and by *Medical Hypotheses*, which published it. It is unlikely this is the only instance of such editorial bias.

Approximately seventy-five percent of clinical research published in the leading medical journals is funded by pharmaceutical companies and medical device manufacturers.[22] Clinical studies that are commercially sponsored have a 5.3 times greater ratio of demonstrating a positive effect of the study agent than do non-commercially sponsored research projects.[23,24] Not only do the clinical researchers have a conflict of interest between their corporate sponsorship and scientific objectivity, but the journals may also have a conflict of interest. Lexchin and Light noted the conflict that journals have with their commercial advertisers.[25] They used the example of the *Annals of Internal Medicine*, which courageously published an article that critically examined the accuracy of pharmaceutical ads and subsequently suffered a loss of advertising revenue in retaliation.[26] Editors of leading medical journals have developed a uniform disclosure form for revealing conflict of interests.[27] This is certainly a step in the right direction, but is not likely to change matters substantially due to the political and economic power of the companies in question.

In a landmark study on the truthfulness and accuracy of medical research, Redman et al.,[28] noted that 325 articles that were retracted had been cited 9,942 times before the retractions occurred and 4,501 times after the retractions occurred. The advancing edge of medical knowledge is indeed more jagged than expected.

Steen observed in a series of articles that 788 articles have been retracted in the past decade and noted that both fraud and error are common causes of retractions.[29] Of note the USA led in publishing articles that were then retracted. I suspect that postmodern lack of moral sensibility underlies this tendency to deceive. Also the large economic consequences of medical discoveries has added to the postmodern "fluidity of fact." Medical research has become a high stakes economic endeavor that encourages a "fudging" of the facts at times. Neither economists nor business executives invented the thinness of the postmodern valuing of integrity, although they may contribute to it. It is a cultural phenomenon and as such it pertains to the cultural values of the entire society. Moral relativism is a social problem in the postmodern

world that involves breakdown in communication, consensus, and valida-
tion.[30]

It should not be a surprise that pharmaceutical companies, most of which
are publicly traded, prioritize profit maximization over scientific objectivity.
They see their first duty to the company and shareholders. Merck's debacle
with Vioxx resulted in reducing, at least temporarily, the stock value. Had the
company pursued a policy of full disclosure of adverse side effects, that
would have minimized the negative impact.

Marcia Angell, a former editor of *The New England Journal of Medicine*
who has written very cogently on this subject, recommends the establishment
of a new federal agency, an "Institute for Prescription Drug Trials,"[31] to
combat industry abuses. Unfortunately, it is difficult to imagine that with the
political climate in Washington and the very substantial lobbying clout of the
pharmaceutical industry that such an agency will ever be established. Idealis-
tically we should focus on ways to reestablish ethical norms within postmodern society rather than solely placing our reliance on legislation and accompanying penalties. However, the postmodern ethos does not foster the sudden
flourishing of ethical norms. More will be elaborated on this in later chapters.

Another important and related concern is the fact that almost two-thirds
of experts that participate in the development of practice guidelines have
financial ties to pharmaceutical companies.[32] Hence it is fair for the healthcare stakeholders (patients, physicians, insurers, and others) to ask how objective and scientific are the practice guidelines of evidence-based medicine,
if they are based on clinical research sponsored by an industry with an
interest in more products that increase their profits, written by experts that
have financial ties. Answers to that question come from Matthew Wynia,
then Director of the Institute for Ethics at the American Medical Association,
and David Boren.[33] They note that there are innumerable methods that an
industry sponsor can use to manipulate a clinical trial to make it likely that
the results will be favorable to their product. These techniques include use of
inappropriate dosing in the comparison drug,[34] not reporting undesirable
clinical endpoints,[35] and inappropriate conduct of clinical trials.[36] They mention that a succession of scandals have already occurred, but that there have
not been any significant regulatory changes to prevent further instances.

Poses states that postmodernists have argued that RCTs became pre-eminent not because they are immune to bias, but because advocates for RCTs
became politically dominant among clinical investigators and funding agencies.[37] I think there is quite a bit of evidence supporting that contention.
Hence, medical research becomes an excellent example of the argument that
knowledge is socially constructed. Foucault, aware of the influences of capitalism in the late twentieth century, also saw the effects of earlier sources of
power when writing about medicine in the eighteenth century. This socially
relativistic aspect of medical investigation has remained even as the research

technologies have advanced dramatically. It is more difficult to alter the socially constructed power equation.

Is it realistic to suggest the possibility of a significant change in the cultural ethos? Perhaps not, but this proposition will be considered further in the last two chapters.

PRACTICE GUIDELINES AND THEIR DISCONTENTS

Inasmuch as practice guidelines are developed from the available knowledge of clinical trials, and that those trials and their publication are subject to power relationships and viewpoints of the sponsors, researchers, reviewers, and editors of the publication, then any guideline will have some degree of subjectivity. On those rare occasions when I have had some direct involvement in the process of advancing a medical discipline's knowledge, I have noticed that these processes resembled other human endeavors in their interdependency with human power relationships. For example, it had become a fairly common clinical practice among clinical nephrologists in the 1980s to prescribe deferroxamine to hemodialysis patients suffering from aluminum overload, a condition characterized by bone disorders and neurologic disorders. Nephrologists were following the advice of experts like Malluche.[38] I became concerned about this particular practice because the manufacturer's drug information indicated that deferroxamine was contraindicated in renal failure. Then I observed two patients who developed a very rare life threatening fungal infection called mucormycosis while receiving deferroxamine.[39] It got a little testy when I questioned this practice at a national conference where the experts were still lecturing on the benefits of deferroxamine. Fortunately, other nephrologists were making similar observations to my own, and this clinical practice was abandoned shortly thereafter. Power relationships may dominate the decision-making for some time but eventually the factual inputs become manifest. Whether and when the facts are heeded is another matter.

Vos, Houtepen, and Horstman[40] suggest modifying the basic Foucauldian insight of power/knowledge in order to consider evidence-based medicine (EBM) as dependent on the relationship between society and government. In addition, they note that epistemology, including medical knowledge, is inherently related to the ordering of the public realm. They go on to say that postmodern culture and thought are not conducive to a single unitary representation of knowledge. They therefore consider EBM as part of a discursive process that involves many stakeholders, and that awareness of the process requires an engaged, informed citizenry. PCORI, by including patients and other healthcare stakeholders, appears to be attempting such an engagement of citizenry in clinical research.[41]

Richardson and Polyakova note that there exists a predilection of medical journals that publish large, expensive studies of clinical interventions that are designed to make substantial profits and that researchers are enmeshed in a web of institutional and professional relationships that dictate the nature of the research that is funded, conducted, and published. [42] Medical knowledge is socially and economically constructed by individuals and corporations motivated to maximize profits because in a postmodern world few values can challenge the primacy of profitability.

An interesting instance of the power/knowledge entanglement occurred when the AHCPR (Agency Health Care Prevention and Research) developed a clinical practice guideline regarding the management of back pain that so upset a powerful group of spine surgeons that they organized a political lobbying effort to eliminate the AHCPR's funding. [43] As a result, the AHCPR suspended its efforts at developing practice guidelines and eventually had to reorganize under another name, the Agency for Healthcare Quality Research (AHRQ). The authors of the original studies that formed the basis for the AHCPR guidelines noted, in an article in *The New England Journal of Medicine*, the need to protect investigators and funding agencies from intimidation by special interests; in this case a particular group of physicians and device manufacturers. [44] Today the AHRQ provides a compendium of practice guidelines developed by *other* healthcare organizations on its website, but does not sponsor development of guidelines itself because of the political danger that it could invoke.

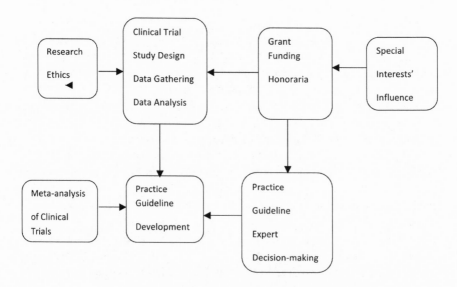

Figure 2.1. Social Construction of Postmodern Medical Knowledge

Another important line of thought is the confluence of the equity principle, socioeconomic status, and evidence-based medicine. Guidelines have
some potential to increase rather than decrease healthcare disparities. Issues
of access, cultural sensitivity, and language translation arise. Aldrich and
associates recommend a four-step process designed to minimize any socioeconomic inequity[45] identifying health interventions, identifying barriers to
such interventions for subpopulations, identifying remedies to the barriers,
and adding them to intervention package.

As an example of such an approach, when I was Chief of General Medicine at the University of Illinois at Chicago my colleagues and I assembled a
multi-disciplinary team that developed a multimedia computerized learning
program for Latino and African American patients on diabetes self-care. We
had some success in crossing language and cultural barriers to reduce healthcare disparities through culturally sensitive education.[46] Specifically, we
were able to increase perceived susceptibility to diabetes complications in the
intervention group with previously poor control. Thus, guidelines need not
increase disparities if sufficient thought and efforts are made in designing
them to include consideration of socio-cultural aspects of implementation.
This is an essential component of ethical conduct regarding practice guidelines in the postmodern era. As Lyotard might state,[47] this is bearing witness
to the *differend*, that pays homage to the outlier by acknowledging the existence and validity of her differing language game.[48]

Some of Lyotard's postmodern thought thoroughly denies the possibility
of an overarching ethic. Paradox and denial of grand narratives are fundamental precepts of postmodern thought. "Just gaming," the phrase that refers
to one of Lyotard's ethical principles, is in itself paradoxical.[49] "Just gaming" implies that there is a plurality of knowledge processes, and that there is
not one dominant process in a knowledge hierarchy There are analogies in
the clinical research realm as I have noted in the preceding discussion. Medical truths are not self-evident and the gaming of medical research and medical publication is not immune to social, political, and economic influences.

Practice guidelines have the potential to enhance clinical care if they are
not implemented in a hegemonic, bureaucratic manner. In some areas such as
the field of anesthesiology[50] and the practice of reducing nosocomial infections,[51] guidelines have already been shown to improve care. However, for
most areas of clinical practice, such clearly delineating evidence is less available. The highly regarded Institute of Medicine issued a report critical of the
guideline development methodology in common use noting substantial evidence of bias in guideline development.[52] Following the Foucaldian insight,
it may be very difficult to remove bias altogether.

It is important that those creating healthcare policy understand that the
texture of clinical practice is not uniform and that a process that works in one
area of clinical medicine may not work in another. How the practice guide-

line committee is constituted will influence the content of the guideline to some extent. Moreover, the corrosive nature of the intrusion of business values in medical practice should not be underestimated. This will be explored further in a later chapter.

IMPLEMENTATION OF GUIDELINES AND PAY FOR PERFORMANCE

The creation of a practice guideline does not ensure that clinicians will follow it. One of the leading implementation processes is found under the recent rubric of "Pay for Performance."[53] In this model, financial incentives are used to promote application of a guideline by rewarding those physicians who comply with it. Such programs require coordination with health insurance plans,[54] and require computerized healthcare information technology. If all insurers are involved in such programs, the financial effect is greater than if only one is involved and raises the stakes. One may consider such an approach an instance of Lyotard's "just gaming" so in some limited sense it may be considered a postmodern version of ethical conduct.

There are several reasons for concern about the efficacy and impact of these incentive programs. A major one is that they tend to measure very small components of care in a systematic manner but fail to account for individual patients' unique characteristics or measure other equally important components of medical care. Such components include an accurate and complete history and physical examination, an appropriate and cost effective diagnostic plan, and a treatment plan that considers biopsychosocial patient aspects as well as biological ones. Patients often have other factors that make them outliers from the study groups that were the evidence basis for the guideline construction. Thus high-quality care requires that the physician understand subgroup analysis and differentiation and can recognize when it is necessary to deviate from the standard because a single approach is not suitable for all patients based on real characteristics.

Another concern is that when a system incorporates the need to pay physicians extra to perform appropriate care, such an approach undermines the professional ethic of doing the correct process out of a sense of duty and responsibility. Even so, it may be necessary to acknowledge that such financial rewards are needed in the postmodern ethos of the twenty-first century. If postmodernism implies little deontological legitimacy, then a postmodern ethic may need to embrace financial rewards in the manner of "just gaming." While I do not favor this approach it may well be needed.

Yet significant pitfalls to this approach have already been identified. Powell et al. reported regarding the VA hospital experience with unintended consequences of a performance measurement system with financial implications.[55] They observed that trying to meet the performance metrics resulted in inappropriate clinical care, excessive polypharmacy, reduced attention to patient concerns, compromises to patient education and autonomy, and adverse impact on the primary care team dynamics and interpersonal relationships. This hardly sounds like a process improvement in clinical care. It sounds more like "unjust gaming," an ironic postmodern twist.

Werner and McNutt question the current approach of applying national guidelines and suggest that local approaches through local collaboratives may prove more fruitful.[56] They did not explain the basis of regional differences fully but I suspect their motivation is to retain some regional control over the regulatory process. They also note that the current approach of quality improvement tends to stifle innovation, and recommend adopting a reward system that involves participation in local or regional improvement collaboratives. This approach sounds more communitarian but also has features of "just gaming" as well. It requires playing with certain rules in place to elicit improved techniques of improvement itself. Such an approach merits further exploration.

Rose notes that there exists a great deal of outside influence in the Pay-for-Performance measurement process[57] with potential for conflicts of interest. He mentions that a leading quality measure development organization, the National Committee for Quality Assurance (NCQA), is heavily sponsored by pharmaceutical companies. Moreover, he points out that professional societies that often devise practice guidelines in their disciplines also have financial ties to the industry. This evokes once again Foucault's admonition that one cannot extract power relationships from the development of knowledge. There may be no practice guideline development without some organization having an interest in influencing the content of the guideline developed. Would a guideline that was entirely funded through the federal government be free of power relationships? Certainly not, but it may favor restraint in spending instead of the current balance which favors profits and resultant excessive healthcare spending.

Consider some of the insights from David Eddy, one of the founding leaders of the quality improvement movement who helped the NCQA develop measurements. He states: "As for inaccuracy, it can creep into performance measurement through every pore. Some of the most obvious sources are insufficient sample sizes, inaccuracies in data sets, the presence of confounding factors that are either understood but not adjusted for or not understood at all."[58] Eddy also points out that evidence-based medicine (EBM) has two distinctive categories: evidence-based guidelines and evidence-based individual patient-based decision-making,[59] with the latter requiring individual physicians to exert their clinical judgment informed by the particular characteristics of a patient as well as the existing body of clinical information.

I advise caution regarding the potential for quality measurements to focus on the easiest quantified measure while ignoring truly monumental factors in quality excellence. Such excellence includes accurate diagnosis and tailoring patient care to individual patient characteristics. Researchers from the Rand Corporation note that the results of clinical trials are frequently ambiguous, rarely yield definitive results that can be adopted uniformly for a broad population, and are frequently misconstrued.[60] Is guideline-based, computerized, bureaucratic medical practice outrunning the science and evidence?

SUMMARY

Only future research will be able to fully assess the benefits and costs of a technologically reliant, standardized approach to healthcare that evidence-based medicine, practice guidelines and computerized order sets with decision support have come to represent. It may be difficult to imagine that there will not be some benefit to such an approach given the pervasive and successful computerization of non-medical human activities. But the cost may be not merely financial, but one that changes the ethos and cultural values of clinical practice in the direction of rote performance of a nationally accepted bureaucratic standard. Whether that standard is driven by industry or the Federal government, the diminished role for the physician's clinical judgment is likely to be an effect of such a development. Such an approach raises serious ethical concerns, one of the most important of which is "unjust gaming" or deciding which interests and influences assert their power to influence the development and composition of evidence-based medical practice.

Even in postmodern times, overarching myths tend to develop and span disparate communities via the Internet and other media. While Lyotard may have announced the end of such meta-narratives, several still lurk in the popular culture. It would be more useful to acknowledge their existence and actively take them into account in devising healthcare policy as well as other public policies.

Richard Rorty, considering Dewey's notion of social hope, spoke of "the need to create new ways of being human."[61] Perhaps we need to aspire to develop new rules of "just gaming" so we create a culturally acceptable manner of practicing ethical medicine in the twenty-first century. My vision of how this can be done is still incomplete but making our cultural myths explicit seems to be an important step in the process.

NOTES

1. Staudenmaier J. M. The atrophy of civic commitment in *Beyond Individualism* ed. Gelpi DL. Univ Notre Dame Press, 1989, p. 144.

2. Foucault M. *The Birth of the Clinic: An Archeology of Medical Perception.* New York: Vintage 1973, p. 197.

3. Cruise J. History of medicine: The metamorphosis of scientific medicine in the ever-present past. *Am J Med Sci* 318(3): 171–184, 1999.

4. Foucault M. *The Birth of the Clinic: An Archeology of Medical Perception.* New York: Vintage 1973, p. 49.

5. Foucault M. *Surveiller et punir.* Paris, Gallimard, 1975, p. 32.

6. Foucault M., ed. Gordon C. *Power/Knowledge: Selected Writings 1972–1977.* New York: Pantheon, 1980, p. 178.

7. Foucault M. *The Archeology of Knowledge.* Trans. A.S. London: Pantheon 1972.

8. Sheridan A. *Michel Foucault: The Will to Truth.* London: Tavistock, 1980, p. 99.

9. Maseide P. The deep play of medicine: Discursive and collaborative processing of evidence in medical problem solving. *Communication Med* 3(1): 43–54, 2006.

10. Polanyi M. *Personal Knowledge: Toward a Post-Critical Philosophy.* London: Routledge & Kegan Paul, 1958, p. 89.

11. Reinders H. The importance of tacit knowledge in practices of care. *J Intellect Disab Res* 54 (suppl 1): 28–37, 2010.

12. Ibid.

13. Freidson E. *Professionalism: The Third Logic.* Chicago: Univ Chicago Press 2001.

14. Reinders H. The transformation of human services. *J Intellect Disab Res* 52(7): 564–572, 2008.

15. Patsopoulos N. A. A pragmatic view of pragmatic trials. *Dialogues Clin Neurosci* 13: 217–224, 2011.

16. Horn S. D., Gassaway J. Practice based evidence: Incorporating clinical heterogeneity and patient-reported outcomes for comparative effectiveness fesearch. *Medical Care* 48(6 suppl1): S17–S22, 2010.

17. Brass E. P. The gap between clinical trials and clinical practice: The use of pragmatic clinical trials to inform regulatory decision making. *Clin Pharmcol. Therapeutics* 87(3): 351–355, 2010.

18. Personal communication PCORI Communications Director, Bill Silberg March 20, 2013.

19. Hayward R. A., Kent D. M., Vian S., Hofer T. P. Reporting clinical trial results to inform providers, payers, and consumers: The need to assess benefits and harms for lower vs high risk patients. *Health Affairs* 24: 1571–1581, 2005.

20. Johnson J. A. Pharmacogenetics: potential for individualized drug therapy through genetics. *Trends Genetics* 19 (11): 660–666, 2003.

21. Eiser A. R. Does Over-expression of Transforming Growth Factor beta account for the increased morbidity in African-Americans: Possible Clinical Study and Research Implications. *Medical Hypotheses.* 75(5): 418–421, 2010.

22. House of Commons Health Committee. *Influence of the Pharmaceutical Industry.* Volume 1. April 22, 2005.

23. Bodenheirmer T. Uneasy Alliance-Clinical Investigators and the pharmaceutical industry. *N Engl J Med* 342: 1539–1544, 2000.

24. Abramson J., Starfield B. The Effect of Conflict of Interest on Biomedical Research and Clinical Practice Guidelines: Can We Trust the Evidence in Evidence Based Research. *JABFP* 18(5): 414–418, 2005.

25. Lexchin J., Light D. W. Commercial influence and the content of medical journals. *BMJ* 332: 1444-1446,2006.

26. Altman L. K. Insidem Medical Journal, a Rising Quest for Profits. *New York Times* August 24, 1999, sect F 7.

27. Drazen J. M., de Leeuw P. W., Laine C., et al. Toward More Uniform Disclosure: The Updated ICMJE Conflict of Interest Report Form. *Ann Intern Med* 153: 268–269, 2010.

28. Redman B., Yarandi H. M., Merz J. F. Empirical developments in retraction. *J Med Ethics* 34: 807–9, 2008.

29. Steen R. G. Retractions in the medical literature: How many patient are put at risk by flawed research. *J Med Ethics* 10: 1136 2011; 37: 113–117.

30. Seidman S. *Postmodern Social Theory as Narrative in Postmodernism & Social Theory*. Ed. Seidman S., Wagner D. G. Blackwell: Oxford, 1992, 47–81.

31. Angel M. *The Truth about Drug Companies: How They Deceive Us and What to Do About It*. New York: Random House, 2004.

32. Choudhry N. K., Stelfox, Detsky A. S. Relationships between authors of clinical practice guidelines and the pharmaceutical industry. *JAMA* 287: 612–617, 2002.

33. Wynia M., Boren D. Better Regulation of Industry-Sponsored Clinical Trials Is Long Overdue. *J Law, Med, Ethics* 37: 410–419, 2009.

34. Brody H. *Hooked: Ethics, the Medical Profession and the Pharmaceutical Industry*. Lanham: Rowman & Littlefield, 2007, p. 342.

35. Durfman G. D., Morrisey S., Drazen J. M. Expression of Concern Reaffirmed. *N Engl J Med* 354(11):1193, 2006.

36. Rennie D., Flanagan A. Authorship, Guests, Ghosts, Grafters, and the Two Sided coin. *JAMA* 271(6):469–471, 2006.

37. Poses R. M. A cautionary tale: The dysfunction of American health care. *Eur J Int Med* 2003 14(2): 123-130.

38. Malluche H. H., Smith A. J., Abreo K., Faugere M. C. The use of deferoxamine in the management of aluminum accumulaton in bone in patients with renal failure. *NEJM* 311(3): 140–44, 1984.

39. Eiser A. R., Neff M. S., Slifkin R. F. Intestinal mucormycosis in hemodialysis patient following deferroxamine. *Am J Kidney Diseases* 1987, 10:71–3.

40. Vos, Houtepen, and Horstma. Evidence based medicine and power shifts in health care systems. *Health Care Analysis* 2002; 10:319–328.

41. PCORI website: http://www.pcori.org/about-us/. Accessed March 20, 2013.

42. Richardson E. T., Polyakova A. The illusion of scientific objectivity and the death of the investigator. *Eur J Clin Invest* 42: 213–215, 2011.

43. Deyo R. A., Psaty B. M., Simon G., Wagner E. H., Omenn G. S. The Messenger Under Attack: Intimidation of Researchers by Special Interest Groups. *N Engl J Med* 336(16): 1176–1179, 1997.

44. Ibid.

45. Aldrich B., Kemp L., Williams J. S., Harris E. et al. Using socioeconomic evidence in clinical practice guidelines. *Brit Med J* 327:1283–1285, 2003.

46. Gerber B. S., I. G. Brodsky, K. A. Lawless, L. I. Smolin, A. M. Arozullah, E. V. Smith, M. L. Berbaum, P. S. Heckerling, A. R. Eiser. Implementation and Evaluation of a Low-Literacy Diabetes Education Computer Multimedia Application. *Diabetes Care* 28(7): 56–63, 2005.

47. Lyotard J. F. *The Differend: Phrases in Dispute*. G. Van Den Abbeele, trans. Minneapolis: Univ Minn Press, 1991.

48. Nuyen A. T. Lyotard's postmodern ethics and information technology. *Ethics Inform Tech* 6: 185–191, 2004.

49. Lyotard J. F., Thiebaud J. L. *Just Gaming*. Godzich W. transl. Minneapolis: Minnesota Univ Press, 1985.

50. Committee on Standards and Practice Parameters, American Society of Anesthesiologists. Practice Guidelines for Post-Anesthesia Care. *Anesthesiology* 96: 742–52, 2002.

51. Bratzler D. W., Houck P. M. Antimicrobial prophylaxis for surgery. *Am J Surgery* 189(4): 395–404, 2005.

52. Institute of Medicine. *Clinical Practice Guidelines We Can Trust*. Washington, DC: Academies Press, 2011, p. 92–94.

53. Epstein A. M. Pay for performance at the tipping point. *N Engl J Med*. 356(5): 515–517, 2007.

54. Mandel K. E., Kotagal U. R. Pay for Performance Alone Cannot Drive Quality. *Arch Pediatr Adolesc Med* 161(7):650–655, 2007.

55. Powell A. A, White K. M, Partin M. R. et al. Unintended consequences of implementing a national performance measurement system into local practice. *J Gen Int Med* 27(4): 405–12, 2011.

56. Werner R. M, McNutt R. A New Strategy to Improve Quality. *JAMA* 301(13): 1375–1377, 2009.

57. Rose J. Industry Influence in the Creation of Pay-for-Performance Quality Measures. *Q Manage Health Care* 17(1): 27–34, 2008.

58. Eddy D. M. Performance Measurement: Problems and Solutions. *Health Aff* 17(4): 7–26, 1998.

59. Eddy D. M. Health Technology Assessment and Evidence-Based Medicine: What are We Talking About? *Value In Health* 12 (supp 12) S6–S7, 2009.

60. Thimbie J. W., Fox D. S., Busum K. V., Schneider E. C. Five reasons that many comparative effectiveness studies fail to change patient care and clinical practice. *Health Affairs*. 31(10): 2168–74, 2012.

61. Rorty R. *Philosophy and Social Hope*. London: Penguin, 1999, p. 88.

Chapter Three

The Culture of Medical Practice

Corporate Computerization versus the Face of the Other

"It is a moral practice that makes caregivers, and at times even the care-receivers, more present and thereby fully human." —Arthur Kleinman[1]

"Increasingly, the central question is becoming who will have access to the information these machines must have in storage to guarantee that the right decisions are made." —Jean-Francois Lyotard[2]

"The relation with the Other, or Conversation, is a non-allergic relation, an ethical relation; but inasmuch as it is welcomed this conversation is a teaching." —E. Levinas[3]

Culture in America is complex and multifaceted so the interaction between culture and medical practice is a tangled web of relationships. Kleinman et al. noted that American allopathic physicians generally disregard both the patient's experience of illness[4] and its personal meaning to the patient in favor of a scientific/technological paradigm. In this paradigm, the physician focuses on diagnosing, treating, and seeking a cure to the ailment or, when a cure is not possible, alleviating the disease process and related symptoms. This lack of sensitivity to the patient's experiences of illness is intensified by differences in ethnicity, cultural background, educational background, and socioeconomic status. Two additional forces have made medical practice more insensitive to the human experience of illness: a greater reliance on a burgeoning and profitable medical technology, and the bureaucratic drive to standardize medical care in an industrial model. What within our medical culture or the larger cultural milieu assures that real change will not occur? Around the time of Kleinman's seminal article, the new "Medical-Industrial

Complex" model of healthcare delivery was also taking shape as aptly described by Arnold Relman.[5] The for-profit medical industry endorsed and accentuated a style of medical practice focused on technological diagnosis and treatment including medical imaging, laboratory testing, prescription medications, and "minimally" invasive surgical and medical procedures. Physicians and other healthcare providers were drawn, along with the increasingly powerful corporations, into the "money vortex of the economy."[6] This rolling out of the overriding business model of healthcare delivery took firm root in the 1980s and its growth continues to accelerate. Fueled by the need to raise capital for hospital expansion and new technology, giant corporations such as Columbia-HCA[7] grew to have dominant roles. Such organizations are led by healthcare executives trained in business schools and rooted in a business ethos rather than a medical one. This ethos aided by rapid technological advancements in medical sciences, the pharmaceutical industry, and other biotechnology industries has brought forth change in the culture of medical care delivery. While the growth of technology produced such remarkable advances as cardiac pacemakers, cochlear implants, implantable catheters for chemotherapy, and numerous other inventions,[8] such growth also had downsides. Much of the clinical research in America today is financed by pharmaceutical companies and medical device companies[9] so it is not surprising that the results of clinical research advances the marketing of the healthcare industry's most expensive products, and that the distinction between research and marketing have been blurred. Academic physicians who have a role in practice guidelines often have a "cozy" relationship with industry.[10] Furthermore, industry representatives showered honorariums upon selected physicians who would speak on topics beneficial to their products and provided other benefits such as "educational" junkets and other marketing related giveaways. Only fairly recently has the Accrediting Council for Continuing Medical Education (ACCME) enacted rules that have substantially impeded such promotions in the form of continuing medical education.[11] So the business culture of medicine has been multi-faceted and overbearing in its intrusion into the medical profession and has impacted virtually every specialty albeit to varying degrees. The professionalism of medicine is its core values of accountability, responsibility for clinical care, integrity, confidentiality, quality, competency, and advocacy for patients.[12] These values require attention to individual human narratives, both biologic and social. However, the business of medicine has fractured that value domain, and replaced it with the business values of return on investment, market share, profitability, and performativity. Lyotard noted: "every profession is in danger of collapsing when another end is imposed upon it, . . . a hegemonic end even if it is only appended to it."[13]

How well have the traditional values of medicine withstood the onslaught of corporate healthcare? How has postmodern culture altered the clinical

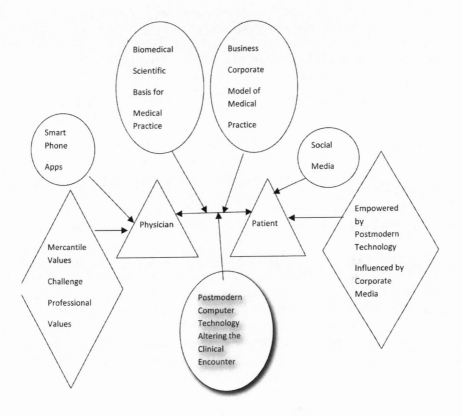

Figure 3.1. Computerized Culture of Postmodern Medicine

encounter? These are not unrelated questions because the postmodern corporation is a crucial determinant of culture, probably the overriding one. Surely one of the manifestations of postmodern consumerism is direct-to-the-consumer medical advertising: an ad for the latest and greatest (and most expensive) treatment, for example: a) improving erectile dysfunction; b) treating rheumatoid and psoriatic arthritis;[14] c) getting a gender-specific knee replacement so that the patient petitions the medical practioner for the product that interests them.[15] This aggressive marketing of medical products is designed to generate more profits although the advertisements promise improvements in many personal aspects of life. No doubt there have been some genuine improvements such as the monoclonal antibodies against tumor necrosis factor in rheumatoid and psoriatic arthritis[16] and the other products advertised but there have also been less efficacious agents equally aggressively marketed. For example, the pain reliever Vioxx, which was removed from the market[17] following revelation of adverse side effects, was also aggressively marketed. Are these advertising campaigns paragons of post-modern information flow or simply shrewd marketing? Both may be the case. Since the manufacturers are no longer permitted to spend extravagantly to "educate" clinicians, they can now put their marketing budget toward beaming the information directly to patients, accompanied by beautiful images of personal fulfillment while the voice-over describes serious unpleasant side effects that are "hopefully" ignored in favor of the beautiful visual images. The advertisers expect humans, being more visual, to ignore those uncomfortable or dangerous side effects but retain those beautiful images and schedule an appointment to implore the physician to prescribe the wondrous medication or request the advertised device, costly as they may be. How does that influence the clinical encounter? The information power relationship has shifted the initiative from the physician to the patient in such instances of advertised medical products, particularly when combined with the influence of patient satisfaction ratings. If the touted agent is neither the best treatment for the patient or on his insurance company's formulary, then the physician has to explain the reasons for not choosing that treatment. Denying a patient the advertised product will probably be viewed unfavorably by the patient. Nearly all physicians are subject to satisfaction ratings by their patients. The power equation in the clinical encounter has hence shifted by the combination of direct to patient advertising and patient satisfaction ratings. How is a layperson going to separate the accurate information from the marketing when it can be difficult for a clinician to do so? The power equation in the clinical encounter now includes pharmaceutical and device manufacturers and their marketing efforts as well as the clinical science, technology, patient advocacy, insurance companies, government, consumerist values, and a variety of inter-personal, corporate, regulatory, and epistemological and phenomenological concerns. Medical care derives not only from biological sciences but also social phenomena including power, politics, and electronic marketing.

While information on the Internet has had a most profound effect in this regard,[18] television has retained considerable potency as well. Television viewing still maintains its status as the electronic media that is most used by the American public.[19] It can be a potent source of medical information. Even my then 90-year-old mother-in-law noticed information on the television news regarding calcium supplements increasing the risk of cardiac disease[20] before I had a chance to read it online or in a journal. (I needed to retreat quickly to my computer to catch up with this publication and attempt to recover some credibility with her.) Hartzband and Groopman[21] note that some patients benefit from Internet information while others are frightened by the undigested information without the guidance of a professional. They also note that health systems have added to the information overexposure by providing patients web access to pathology, laboratory, and radiology reports again without the guidance of a professional. These report results have the potential to be seriously misconstrued by laypersons (and even by professionals). Now the Centers for Medicare and Medicaid (CMS) is demanding that such difficult-to-understand information be conveyed directly to patients.[22] So the clinical encounter is characterized by a more egalitarian information flow but also more angst and entropy as well as more bureaucratic government intervention. Who has not encountered patients bewildered amidst difficult to assess information that is available to them in the name of autonomy? I, for one, have seen it with increasing frequency. The social entropy in our healthcare system is not being reduced by either bureaucratic regulation nor by corporate performativity as they replace older norms of medical professionalism and medical paternalism.

POSTMODERN COMPUTERIZATION AND CONSUMERISM

Lyotard notes that, "computerization becomes the 'dream' instrument for controlling the market system, extended to include knowledge itself."[23] He adds that such effects tend to level hierarchal relationships, as we have observed recently in the medical encounter. But will it improve the clinical encounter if patients feel equal to physicians? Will it help them be compliant with a medical regimen when they are less respectful of a medical professional's recommendations? The narrative of the all-knowing physician is gone and will not be coming back. It was inaccurate at best and overbearing and smug at worst. Many patients and feminists alike are pleased to see such paternalism no longer considered acceptable. Unwelcome pockets of it may remain however. The question remains whether the current physician-patient relationships are improving in this era of burgeoning information technology? Do we need to find a new basis for the patient-physician relationship? Where shall the relational balance be properly reset?

Another blow to physician agency in postmodern culture is the online patient ratings of physicians.[24] The number of sites rating physicians has proliferated, and since individuals who do the posting are not sampled in a statistically valid manner, the results are not necessarily accurate and probably attract outliers in both directions—both the displeased and very pleased. Ratings on some websites also rate plumbers, hairdressers and others. This helps to declassify physicians as a distinctive profession when they are grouped with other services that require considerably fewer years of education and training than physicians as well as a differing set of values (this is not to devalue plumbers and other service trades). The development of online ratings has engendered new enterprises designed to preserve online reputations.[25] Online ratings are a still developing social phenomenon.

Borgmann[26] has observed: "Information technology has become the engine of the postmodern economy" and that, "virtuality is our reply to the devastation of common meanings. Hyperinformation is our response to the oblivion of individuals."[27] Are anonymous postings on a website that lack statistical validity creating valuable information or adding discord to an increasingly fractious clinical milieu? Are such quasi-democratic aspects of the Internet adding to a culture of antagonism?

Thus the power equation is changing and physicians are feeling the effects of this shift. On a leading physician blog, Kevin MD, emergency doctors are noted to complain about being pressured by hospital administrators to readily dispense narcotic pain killers to patients who come in the ED demanding them.[28] The hospital administrators are in turn motivated by patient satisfaction surveys known as *Hospital Consumer Assessment of Healthcare Providers and Systems* (HCAHPS).[29] HCAHPS mandates that all hospitals receiving payments from CMS participate in this survey regularly. CMS publishes the results of these patient surveys on the CMS website, and hospital administrators perceive that these results could influence market share. By exerting such influence on physicians' prescribing of potent, potentially dangerous narcotic drugs, they are following the business dictum that "the customer is always right," but this hardly makes for informed clinical decision-making or safe medical practice. Ostensibly justifiable business practices do not always make for sound medical judgment. Clearly in the clinical realm this intrusiveness of business values can be dangerous to the patient's well-being as well as to the morale of physicians. The latter may not seem so important to the casual observer but it is fundamental if the ethos of a humane professionalism is to be preserved. One cannot expect to regard physicians as merely assiduously trained technocrats and expect that all the values of the medical profession, especially accountability above and beyond the minimum standard, will flourish. A sense of extraordinary service requires a sense of extraordinary accomplishment, and our best clinicians possess both. Postmodern life poses a serious challenge to the pursuit of excellence because it undervalues accomplishment in the grand leveling of values. Foucault stated: "Knowledge derives not from some subject of knowledge but from the power relations that invest it."[30] However, disrupting the power relations is not a guarantee of an improved human condition. Power relations rearrange themselves often in unexpected, contradictory and sometimes unpleasant ways. A blueprint forward is not explicitly apparent.

If information technology is successful in reducing the inequality of the power relationship in clinical medicine, will a less powerful physician be sufficiently motivated and empowered to pursue clinical excellence in practice? Whence comes the emotional motivation to do so? If clinicians are not admired by staff, colleagues, and patients, then medicine becomes reduced to a service for mercantile exchange like any other while admiration and respect recede in the rearview mirror. With the wind forced out of the clinician's sails so to speak, the "disenchantment" of medical practice may well be detrimental to patient and physician alike. This almost certainly has already occurred. When faced with a life-threatening condition, one does not want to be reminded of the fallibility and human frailty of the treating physicians. One hopes one's clinicians have some larger-than-life characteristics, but increasingly they may not. The postmodern non-hero does not inspire the image of the gifted healer. Is there a middle ground without over-dramatizing the two extremes? This middle space needs exploration and does not yield easy answers.

The developing outcomes measurement movement may provide some motivation to perform well. Physicians and other clinical providers do not want to appear below average to themselves or others. However, there are negative emotional implications to such a bureaucratic approach. A combination of the prevailing business ethos, availability of online medical information, and computerization of online physician ratings that are not statistically validated combine to create an uneasy environment for physicians. Now add in the difficulty of dealing with multiple insurance plans motivated to deny payments to physicians and other providers, and the ever-present threat of malpractice litigation. Now the physician is feeling increasingly more like the underdog than the hero even if he or she is part of the select highly compensated surgical and medical specialties. Physicians in those highly compensated disciplines like radiology still command respect from hospital administrators for their revenue generation. A hierarchy exists within the medical profession that is closely linked to reimbursement policies and specialization. The procedurally-focused specialties have maintained some control within this power structure, but they too are threatened by the shifts occuring in reimbursement, mergers and acquisitions, and accountable care organizations (ACOs). ACOs are the latest innovation in medical reimbursement designed to reduce medical costs through the bundling of payments.[31] An ACO is a healthcare provider organization that agrees to contract for healthcare services that have a component of quality measurement and cost consciousness. It places some of the risk of the cost of the care on the provider organization, analogous although not identical to full risk capitation of an earlier managed care era. The business proposition, the clinical care, and the performance metrics are mixed and re-mastered in a postmodern pastiche of communicative capitalism with much flow of information but little if any dialogue. There are many data downloads required in this process but little room for interpersonal communication. Lyotard,[32] citing Luhmann, states that in postmodern societies the normativity of law is succeeded by the performativity of procedures.[33] Performativity in this regard refers to how language usage and rules define and redefine the procedures of healthcare as subservient to the economics of the clinical care. Professionalism and professional regulations have been subsumed beneath the weight of corporate medicine and a consumerist mode of medical practice.

LEVINAS AND THE OTHER IN THE CLINICAL ENCOUNTER

Postmodern thought is not monolithic; it possesses another facet aside from deconstructing modernist myths. Levinas is a postmodern thinker who offers an affirmative ethical experience, the radical encounter of the Other as an ethical force of responsibility. His approach to ethics may offer an important paradigm for the clinical encounter. The unencompassable transcendence of the Other can speak to experience of the patient and clinician, even if only with some difficulty. Dorothy Owens, in *Hospitality to Strangers: Empathy and the Physician-Patient Relationship*, notes that Levinas' notion of the face to face encounter raises the moral claims on the physician when encountering the patient while each maintains his/her distinctive separation. [34]

The ethical priority of the Other: the face to face encounter that elicits the "unencompassable transcendence of the Other evoking the priority of the individual patient's consciousness or "alterity."[35] The epiphany of the Other's face and speech then ruptures the physician's reductionist certainty and invites her to encounter the patient's subjectivity in a powerful experience. The face of the Other commands us to recognize her subjectivity as real and radically different from one's own, yet fully present and of ethical impact. Perhaps this can awaken the physician in an epiphany to the sensibility of the patient as Other. "The Other needs me and calls me and I am ethically obliged to serve her."[36] However in reality, it may be only a small minority of physicians that possesses the sensibility to appreciate the Other in that fashion. A study of oncologists and surgeons treating cancer patients showed that they missed the opportunity to express empathy ninety percent of the time. [37] So while Levinas may provide an exemplary model, few physicians are likely to attain this sensibility without some significant changes in the training milieu or the selection process or a rather substantial change in our culture itself.

Levinas holds that awareness of the Other can overcome cultural limitation and dependence. "To catch sight, in meaning, of a situation that precedes culture, to envision language out of the revelation of the Other . . . in the gaze of a human being looking at another human . . . in the nakedness of his face. . . ."[38]

The face-to-face encounter awakens an epiphanic moment of revelation that entails responsibility and much more. If a physician can experience that moment then she or he can have a true encounter with the patient that transcends cultural differences, business ethos, online ratings, and the other detritus of postmodern life. However, this may be hard to attain for resident physicians steeped in the ethos of postmodern culture replete with expectations of not-so-delayed gratification, limited responsibility, social media, satire, work life/balance, and electronic materialism. Today there may be fewer face to face encounters when the clinician is "locked on" to a computer screen and portions of the evaluative examination are performed by an assistant.

Obligation is immanent once one is aware of it: the ethical being, according to Levinas, initiates the encounter with the face of the Other who elicits an obligation to care (from the physician). The ambiguity of the Other testifies to mystery in the relationship and to the locus of empathy in the "between" as the face of the suffering stranger opens the door to the infinite. The physician needs to feel the humanness and empathy of the patient in reciprocity. If the patient is ungrateful, complaining, and indifferent, the mystical-ethical element of the clinical encounter dissipates, and is replaced by *anomie* in the clinical encounter. Increasingly, this is becoming the more frequent experience of the clinician and patient alike although some encounters are still instilled with the ethos of caring and respect. If the societal ethos follows a consumerist model, eliciting the face of the Other is a fleeting image in the rearview mirror.

Levinas's responsibility for the Other is a challenging model to enact in medical practice, and while I am quite sure Levinas had an extraordinary sensibility for the Other, I am not sure today's clinicians do. Derrida called Levinas's *Totality and Infinity* a treatise on hospitality. Not many physicians conceive of their role in terms of hospitality but rather as purveyors of a scientific-technical craft. Patients are regarded by the industry as consumers and the data-driven business model prevails. Not a fertile milieu for cultivating the moral sensibility, even if one is inclined to do so. Some nurses may be more inclined to consider hospitality part of their mission but they are hardly immune to the corporate business ethos that intrudes on nursing practice as it does on medical practice.

So for the postmodern clinician, one must acknowledge the potential of a Levinasian sensibility for the Other as an exemplary model but then seek a less lofty perch to purse "dialogical sociality" for the clinical encounter. There is much work to be done in developing such middle ground and I will suggest one such approach to establishing a dialogical middle ground.

IMAGINING THE MEDICAL ENCOUNTER AGREEMENT: A HEURISTIC DEVICE

As noted above, not all physicians will feel the face of the Other as described by Levinas. That sensibility is not part of the medical school admission selection process nor does it naturally arise during the medical clerkship or residencies when medical students are engrossed in the mastery of clinical skills, a mountain of medical knowledge, and the intricacies of clinical encounters.[39] Since medical schools still seek students capable of assimilating large quantities of information and reiterating it, one can't count on such students being particularly sensitive or empathic. Humanistic qualities are welcome but not required. There is a considerable spectrum of humanity in the medical profession, whereby some feel the otherness evoked by the face of the Other in its moral voice while several clearly do not. Many fall somewhere between the extremes.

Consider the possibility of the physician and patient entering into a mutual agreement. It may deflect some of the difficulties currently experienced in clinical medicine. Because medicine is a business today administered and led by business men and women it does not create cultural spaces where a dialogic patient-physician encounter can flourish.

Consider such an agreement as a heuristic device for furthering the patient-physician relationship. The basic content of the provider portion in such an agreement can be found on hospital walls throughout the nation, posted to meet federal regulations stating patient rights and responsibilities:

Patient Rights

- Right to be treated with respect
- Right to make treatment choices including refusal of treatment
- Right to obtain access to medical records
- Right to privacy of your medical records
- Right to informed consent in understandable language (including translation)
- Right to make decisions about end-of-life care (complete an advance directive)
- Right to know who to contact when the physician is not available and who will be covering
- Right to receive medical care within the current Standard of Care

The entitlement of patients' rights should be accompanied by patients' responsibilities. In order to get the best care and obtain successful medical outcomes, I am suggesting the list below in the context of "dialogic sociality":

Patient Responsibilities

- Make a reasonable attempt to maintain healthy personal habits
- Be respectful to clinical providers, physicians, nurses, and other providers
- Be honest with healthcare providers

- Comply with diagnostic and treatment plans, and if one cannot, to inform clinicians of areas of non-compliance and, when possible, explain why one could not comply
- Prepare for contingencies, such as running out of medications, so treatment plan is not interrupted
- Make a serious effort to be informed about one's health and health problems to the best of one's ability
- Understand prescription drugs, including side effects, and do not give drugs to other people to use
- Meet financial obligations as best as possible
- Avoid putting others (patients or staff) at risk by following isolation techniques for communicable diseases and not otherwise spreading communicable diseases

Physicians should also make their duties and rights explicit. I suggest the following:

Physician Responsibilities

- Medical competence: knowledgeable of timely medical information and clinical skills in the discipline practiced, i.e., practice evidence-based medical care including seeking appropriate board certification
- Communication competency in keeping the patient and or surrogate decision makers informed of her/his condition, diagnosis, and treatment plan in understandable language
- Treat patients with respect and dignity regardless of race, ethnicity, socioeconomic status, gender, sexual orientation
- Follow professionalism standards and maintain knowledge of medical ethics
- Work with the patient, other healthcare professionals, and staff in a professional fashion to provide the patient with the care that meets or exceeds the standard
- Consult other healthcare professionals when indicated, including use of telehealth when available

Physician Rights

- Be spoken to in a courteous manner
- Receive honest communication from the patient
- Right to not be threatened with bodily or other harm by the patient or family
- Have access to the patient's medical information so informed clinical decisions can be made

• Earn reasonable compensation

Even conceiving of a dialogic pact between patient and healthcare provider is inconsistent with the consumerist model of healthcare which is devoid of any dialogic encounter and candor. Sometimes the phrase "patient-centered care" can be more of a marketing ploy than a reality. Even if patient-centeredness is followed faithfully, I am not sure that eliminates the excesses of the current model of healthcare as a business enterprise.

Of course, today numerous other providers are involved in the care of the patient including nurse practitioners, physician assistants, nurses, physical therapists, pharmacists, dieticians, social workers, health educators, and several others. One could ask where do they fit into this theoretical patient-provider pact? There is no doubt they wish to assert a significant role too.

The postmodern power re-equilibration of the clinical encounter needs a redefining of the "rules of clinical engagement." Maseide notes "Power is made effective through forms of control and methods of domination. . . . As such, they are essential resources of the doctors ability to do his or her work adequately. . . . The impact of power is effective to the extent that the doctor and patient share a system of knowledge and assumptions that facilitate relatively conflict-free interaction and effective patient compliance."[40] But that power dominance relationship has dissipated from many patient-physician interactions, especially those involving primary care physicians. A patient-clinician compact is an effort to establish a more explicit and symmetric relationship and define roles and responsibilities. But in defining responsibilities, why stop with clinicians and patients? Why not ask about the roles and responsibilities of the business executives that usually make key decisions in the healthcare industry? Don't we also need a pact for the healthcare executives and over-reaching bureaucrats of all types, both governmental and private? Make responsibilities explicit for all stakeholders in healthcare.

ALIGNING WHAT PATIENT AND PHYSICIAN VALUE IN THE CLINICAL ENCOUNTER

Several years ago my associates and I came up with the notion that if one could match physician and patient by a set of values in the clinical encounter one could develop a happier clinical dyad. As part of this study, I developed a series of questions to ask both physician and patient that could assess congruence in their decision-making style, desire for information from the clinician, patients' values and religious beliefs, and interest in using herbal remedies.

We completed a study of both internists and family physicians and their patients. The study demonstrated that congruence in clinical values especially information sharing correlated with patient satisfaction.[41] I approached a managed care insurance plan and tried to convince them to implement such patient-physician "matching" by clinical value congruence but so far no insurance plan has tried this approach, perhaps not yet seeing the return on such an effort.

While we have shown that patient satisfaction can improve by matching patient and clinician, it is not improbable that patient outcomes could improve as well through greater compliance with the medical regimen. Moreover there is the opportunity of not merely measuring patient satisfaction but using this instrumental device to "drill down" to how best to match patient and clinician for a productive clinical relationship. We can ask after Lyotard who shall have the access to the information contained in our medical machines and how wisely will they be used, and toward what ends. The advancement of technological information may yield benefits if applied wisely and not be solely focused on return on investment.

SUMMARY

The biomedical model, flawed as it was for not considering the experiential and cultural aspects of medical care, moved more in the direction of a business model than toward an anthropological one as medical practice became fully enmeshed in a burgeoning trillion dollar for-profit industry. Postmodern advertising, as well as information of various types on the Internet altered the power relationships in the clinical encounter and raised uncertainty in the revised relationships. Lyotard's critique of postmodern life and information technology can explain some of the change. Computerization provides a powerful effect on information dispersion as well as on power relationships in the clinical setting. Consumerism encouraged less of a dialogic relationship while the computer posited itself between the faces of the patient and the clinician.

Levinas offers a model of personal encounter with an implicit ethical responsibility for the Other that can be applied to the clinical encounter and could offer an alternative to the old virtue-based model of medical professionalism. However few physicians are likely to automatically possess such a sensibility, being influenced by postmodern culture themselves. I have made some suggested considerations that could bolster the Levinasian ideal:

1) Position the postmodern clinical encounter between patient and clinical care team as a dialogic encounter with rights and responsibilities on both sides.

2) Ask what is the nature of the responsibilities of the business executives that control much of the decision-making in healthcare, both to the patients and the clinical providers?

3) Orchestrate an effort to better match primary care physician to the patient in terms of what values should be considered in the clinical encounter. Postmodern clinical care must be inventive in order to replace what has been lost in the encounter under apparent, probably ineluctable, cultural change. We must nurture new approaches to improve the clinical encounter and not merely bemoan the lost ideals of a bygone era. Some of these approaches may work, improving the clinical encounter for both patient and clinician. It is worthwhile to explore them.

NOTES

1. Kleinman A. On Caregiving. *Harvard Magazine* July 2010.

2. Lyotard J. F. *The Postmodern Condition*. Manchester University Press, 1984. http://www.brainyquote.com/quotes/quotes/j/jeanfranc370945.html

3. Levinas E. *Totality and Infinity: An Essay on Exteriority Transl.* Lingis A. Pittsburgh: Duquesne University Press, 1969.

4. Kleinman A., Eisenberg L., Good B. Culture Illness and Care: clinical lessons from anthropologic and cross-cultural research. *Ann Int Med* 88:251–258, 1978.

5. Relman, A. S. The New Medical-Industrial Complex. *NEJM* 303:963–970, 1980.

6. Ginzberg, Eli. For Profit Medicine: A Reassessment *NEJM* 319:757–761, 1988.

7. Ackman D. The Disaster of the Day: HCA http://www.forbes.com/2000/12/15/1215disaster.html. Accessed July 29, 2011.

8. Healy B. A Medical Industrial Complex. *USNWR* 138 (3); 54 , 2005.

9. Rosman M. Millette K. Bero Metanalysis Trials of Pharmaceutical Treatments.

10. J. Fauber, E. Gabler. Doctors with links to drug companies influence treatment guidelines. *Milwaukee Sentinel Journal*. December 18, 2012.

11. *ACCME*. Essential Areas and their Elements. http://www.accme.org/dir_docs/doc_upload/f4ee5075-9574-4231-8876-5e21723c0c82_uploaddocument.pdf. Revised 2006.

12. Barondess J. Medicine and Professionalism. *Arch Int Med* 163:145–149.

13. Lyotard Jean-Francois. *The Postmodern Explained*. Minneapolis: Univ Minnesota Press, 1993. P64.

14. http://www.enbrel.com/psoriatic-arthritis/psoriatic-arthritis-treatment.jspx?WT.mc_id=paidsearch_Google_phil-+mickelson-+enbrel&WT.srch=1

15. McDonald S., Charron K. D., Bourne R. B. Gender Specific Knee Replacement. Prospective Clinical Outcomes. *Clin Orthop Relat Res.* 2008 November; 466 (11) : 2612–2616. Published online 2008 September 18. doi: 10.1007/s11999-008-0430-1

16. Mease P. J., Goffe B. S., Metz J., et al. Etrarcept in the treatment of psoriatic arthritis and psoriasis: A randomized trial. *Lancet* 356:385–390, 2000.

17. Vioxx voluntary removal from the market. http://www.pbm.va.gov/vioxx/Dear%20Healthcare%20Professional.pdf

18. Gerber B. S., Eiser A. R. The patient physician relationship in the Internet age: Future prospects and the research agenda. *J Med Internet Res.* 3(2):E16, 2001.

19. Television quote in Sachs J.

20. Bolland M. J., Avenell A., Baron J. A., et al. The effects of calcium supplements on the risk of myocardial infarction and cardiovascular effect *BMJ* 2010; 341:c3691 doi: 10.1136/bmj.c3691

21. Hartzband P., Groopman J. Untangling the Web-Patients, Doctors, and the Internet. *NEJM* 362(12): 1063–6, 2010.

22. Freemire J. J., Wieland J. Ober/Kaler Attorneys at Law http://www.ober.com/publications/1518-changes-hipaa-privacy-rule-clia-regs-will-require-laboratories-release. Accessed December 16, 2012.

23. Lyotard J-F. The Postmodern Condition: A Report on Knowledge. University Minnesota Press, 1984 p. 67.

24. Vitals.com http://www.vitals.com/?gclid=CMTbs_utp6oCFeVx5Qodd2uOYw.

25. Bennett, N., & Martin, C. L. (2008, March 10). Corporate reputation—What to do about online attacks: Step no.1: Stop ignoring them. *The Wall Street Journal* .

26. Borgmann A. *Holding-on to Reality*. University of Chicago Press, 1999, p. 4.

27. Ibid., p. 230.

28. Kevin M. D., Commentary on Kevin M. D. http://www.kevinmd.com/blog/2012/02/patient-satisfaction-kill.html

29. HCAHPS Hospital Care Quality from the Consumer Perspective http://www.hcahpsonline.org/home.aspx.

30. Sheridan, Alan. *Foucault: The Will to Knowledge*. Routledge, 2004, 216.

31. Accountable Care Organizations. https://www.cms.gov/ACO/.

32. Lyotard J. F. *The Postmodern Condition: A Report on Knowledge*. University Minnesota Press, 1984, p. 46.

33. Luhrmann N. *Legimation durch Verfahren*. Neuwald: Luchterhand, 1969.

34. Owens Dorothy M. *Hospitality to Strangers: Empathy and the Physician-Patient Relationship*. 1999 Atlanta: Scholars Press p. 79.

35. Levinas E. *Alterity and Transcendence*. Transl. M. B. Smith. Columbia University Press NY, 1999.

36. Clifton-Soderstrom M. Levinas and the Patient as Other: The Ethical Foundation of Medicine. *J Med Phil* 28(4): 447–460, 2003.

37. Morse D., Edwardsen E. A., Gordon H. S. Missed opportunities for interval sympathy in lung cancer communication. *Arch Int Med* 168(17): 1853–1858, 2008.

38. Levinas E. *Basic Philosophical Writings*. Ed. Peperzak, Critchely S., Brenasconi R. Indianapolis: Indiana Univ Press, 1996, p. 58.

39. Neumann, M., Edelhäuser, F., Tauschel, D., Fischer, M.R., Wirtz, M., Woopen, C., Haramati, A., Scheffer, C. Empathy Decline and Its Reasons: A Systematic Review of Studies with Medical Students and Residents. *Academic Medicine*. 86.8: 996–1009, 2011. http://www.ncbi.nlm.nih.gov/pubmed/21670661.

40. Massaide P. Possibly abusive, often benign, always necessary. On power and domination in medical practice. *Sociol Health Illness* 13:545–561, 1991.

41. Schwartz A., Hussain M., Eiser A. R., Lincoln E., Elstein A. Patient-Physician Fit: An Exploratory Study of a Multidimensional Instrument. *Med Decis Making* 26:122–133, 2006.

Chapter Four

Practical and Ethical Concerns Regarding Aspects of Quality Improvement Measures

"Many people recognize that technology often comes with unintended and undesirable consequences." —Leon Kass[1]

"There is no power relation without the correlative constitution of a field of knowledge, nor any knowledge that does not presuppose and constitute at the same time power relations." —M. Foucault[2]

The quality improvement movement has generated several genuine and substantial improvements in healthcare delivery by introducing methodologies that apply the techniques of statistical quality control for reducing medical errors while creating greater awareness of the causes of errors including faulty processes, poor communications, and failure to follow policies.[3,4] Many diverse stakeholders are interested in and value efforts to improve the quality of healthcare including accrediting agencies such as the Joint Commission, insurers, hospitals, healthcare systems, employers, patient groups as well as healthcare providers and their professional societies. Quality improvement initiatives are crucial and will remain an integral and important part of healthcare delivery in the twenty-first century. Yet the nature and context of healthcare delivery and its related technologies are varied and complex so that the efforts to improve quality can have unintended, less salutary consequences. This chapter examines some of those unintended, less sanguine effects. The four areas of concern are: transparency of physician specific process and outcomes measures; the emphasis by healthcare organizations on minimizing variance in clinical practice; the effects of outcomes measures on health disparities among vulnerable populations; and the aspect

49

of practice guidelines that involves their social construction. I examine these matters in the context of the classical bioethical precepts of justice, autonomy, beneficence, and non-malfeasance, as well as through postmodern reflections.

ETHICAL IMPLICATION OF TRANSPARENCY

One aspect of the quality improvement movement in healthcare is the increasing transparency of measured outcomes and processes for individual physicians much as it has been done for hospitals. The most widely discussed examples today are the Pay-for-Performance programs (P4P) that various health insurance plans, including the "core measures" that the Center for Medicare and Medicaid Services (CMS) have implemented as well as Healthcare Effectiveness Data and Information Set (HEDIS) indicators of the National Committee for Quality Assurance (NCQA). The NCQA accredits health insurance plans, practices, and provider organizations.[5] Success by these standards can impact reimbursement rates, marketing of healthcare services, and other aspects of medical practice.

Conclusions regarding quality of care based on computerized data collection may, however, be misleading for several reasons. These include limits on the accuracy of data available from an electronic health record, the very limited scope of the data used in quality measures, and the lack of correction for confounding factors, including patient factors regarding outcomes. For example, a patient may experience a venous thromboembolism after an orthopedic procedure and then have a distinct hospitalization on a hospitalist service.

There is a tendency to attribute accuracy to digitally stored data but such data may have been recorded inaccurately or corrupted during a downloading process. Moreover, the data from individual providers may lack statistical significance because of small sample size for a particular parameter, failure to correct for confounding factors, or errors in data collection and entry. Even when correction factors are known, they may not be applied to a physician's sample because the database lacks the robustness to apply an adjustment factor. Moreover, patients today are generally cared for by several clinicians simultaneously in different disciplines, so identifying a specific physician with a particular process or outcome is often difficult if not impossible. The databases commonly used lack the technical detail to distinguish precisely which provider was responsible for a particular outcome. Outcomes also may be attributable to patient characteristics including compliance,[6] whether the insurer provided access to the needed diagnostic and treatment interventions in a timely manner or not, and other factors unrelated to the quality of care rendered by the clinician.

Another issue is what gets measured may be the factor most easily measured rather than what is most important in clinical care. As Casalino, a leading expert in the field of quality measurement noted, "what doesn't get measured may be a greater indicator of quality than what does get measured."[7] This is so because of the complexity of medical diagnosis, the varied texture of both the illness and the communication of symptoms, and the interaction between general principles gleaned from clinical trials and the applications to individual patients who may have significant factors causing them to differ from a group studies in a randomized clinical trial. Thygeson et al. note that "Randomized controls trials are the evidentiary standard for medical truth. They are designed to study biological systems in the laboratory, not social systems in the real world."[8] Medical care is rendered in the social systems that occur in real world conditions so we have set up a standard of medical truthfulness that may not serve all patients as well as the "ideal median" patients who serve as subjects of clinical trials.

If measures of specific physicians are inaccurate but construed as valid and made public, then the precept of justice is violated. The principle of justice calls for an accuracy of evaluation that current techniques may simply not be capable of. While quality improvement researchers recognize their discipline's shortcomings and limitations, bureaucrats that create policy may not comprehend the nuanced nature of the measurement discipline. Hence they may create policy that lacks both statistical validity and just conclusions about the quality of the care rendered by clinical providers.

In a review of Pay-for-Performance studies, Peterson et al.[9] noted instances of improved documentation rather than improved performance and reduced access for the sickest patients who may reduce a physician's and a hospital's performance on the measures. Both of these findings raise ethical concerns regarding the potential for the gaming of the measurements to the detriment of the sickest of patients. For example, clinicians may seek to drop the sickest and least compliant patients from their panel in order to improve their outcomes measures. In fact, there is recent evidence that this is occurring.[10] If measurements of care disadvantage the sickest or most vulnerable of patients, that would be a violation of the precepts of justice and beneficence by reducing the access to appropriate care for the most challenging patients. This is a potentially serious unintended consequence of the ratings being increasingly implemented in today's bureaucratized clinical practice. Seeking the best for every patient is a laudable goal but if the quality improvement methods available inadvertently disadvantage the most vulnerable, then the process has not advanced the cause of justice nor beneficence. Apel has noted that science and ethics have gone in disparate directions.[11] Excessive trust in the meaningfulness of computerized quality data may drive ethics and the "science" of quality improvement apart as well if injustice inadvertently occurs.

TRANSPARENCY AND THE PATIENT-PHYSICIAN RELATIONSHIP

The effect of transparency of physician quality measures could be detrimental if it reveals information that impacts the patient-physician relationship negatively while actually impacting the quality of care minimally. For example, if a patient learns that her personal physician's data is below the mean on some measure of one or more of the HEDIS indicators (developed by NCQA to measure quality of primary care), [12] that may reduce a patient's trust in that physician. The greater number of measures taken the greater likelihood that any given clinician will have some parameters below the mean. One can imagine a patient that has had her/his personal physician for several years, but now does not have the same trust in her because of knowledge of some below- average indicator (one always tends to *assume* that one's personal physician is above average). The patient may stay with this physician but not listen to her/his advice or may leave the practice. The patient may seek to change to a physician with top scores, only to discover that such physicians in the area are not taking new patients. Is that patient better off knowing her physician's scorecard, if all it does is create turbulence in the patient-physician relationship? Does data transparency trample on the ongoing patient-physician relationship? One could refer to this phenomenon as the negative "Lake Wobegon" effect wherein every patient desires an above average physician although half the physicians are below average at least on some measured parameter. Disclosure of such information, by damaging the patient-physician relationship, violates the precept of non-malfeasance because harm is done by disclosing such information.

Treating medical care strictly as a measurable commodity may be dangerous to one's health as well as to healthcare providers' reputations and morale if inaccuracy and inexactitude of the data are misleading and unnecessarily impugn the quality of the care they render.

Is the computerized information even accurate or was an inappropriate sample used to assess the parameter? In outcomes measurements by organizations, as distinguished from those by outcomes researchers, rigorous rules of statistical validity are not always observed with regard to sampling size or case mix adjustment for confounding factors.

A recent RAND study demonstrated the inaccuracy of administrative databases for identifying a physician's practice cost profile. [13] There is no reason to think analogous databases for quality measures will be any more accurate.

Woodhandler and Himmelstein raise additional concerns that intensive coding by some clinicians or practices may distort the results as these differences often go undetected. [14] Moreover they raise the legitimate concern that offering financial incentives may undermine the more noble motivations of pursuing clinical excellence and altruistic motives. Financial incentives may be effective at getting a clinician's attention but run the risk of corrupting other motivations as then reinforce consumerist values wherein the physician is a "consumer of work units" as well as a producer of services.

One assuredly can see the value in identifying and remediating poorly performing physicians but current methods of quality measurement may actually not detect them. In addition the majority of physicians, even those in a decile or two below the mean on some limited set of measures may still be quite capable clinicians. Yet knowing the specifics of the measurement scores may not only harm the physicians themselves but also their patients. Moreover, even those physicians below the mean may excel at something even if it is just accessibility, emotional intelligence, or empathizing with the patient which goes unreported in the database. Another approach to "weeding out" or remediating poorly performing physicians may well be needed but it should not be based solely on data downloads. It could include a comprehensive method involving medical directors, department chairs and chief medical officers, individuals who are physicians themselves and familiar with many aspects of the physician's work and are able to take into consideration many factors including the quality outcomes and clinical process data but not limited to them alone. Of course, tort law tends to inhibit the success of such efforts when the tort argument is unlawful restraint of trade against the physician whose privileges are challenged. Ironically lack of tort reform as well as the lack of national licensure standards assure that the least capable physician continues to practice in many instances by moving to another state. The newer Joint Commission regulations regarding focused and ongoing physician review for continued hospital privileges envision a multi-source process that includes chart review, direct observation as well as pre-defined screening criteria, and it recognizes that "most practitioners perform well."[15] These processes have also been challenged to obtain meaningful data.

The principle of non-malfeasance is involved in this matter if harm to the patient-physician relationship occurs without any benefit from revealing process variations that have minimal effect on outcomes. There is also a type of medical Heisenberg uncertainty principle at work in this field. The Heisenberg uncertainty principle in physics states that a particle's position and momentum cannot be measured simultaneously because the measurement itself changes its location and/or momentum.[16] An analogous phenomenon is operative in social systems such as medical practice where the measurements tend to refocus the attention and effort to whatever is measured and remunerated while that which does not get measured receives less attention. No one, in my estimate, would call those items measured in Pay-for-Performance measures a comprehensive assessment of what constitutes quality medical care although the processes may be an important component. There is much

pretense when organizations declare that they are measuring quality compre-
hensively solely with these downloadable measurements. At least one assessment organization performs their assessments without ever visiting the provider by using an electronic database to collect their data for assessment.[17]

TRANSPARENCY CAN BE GOOD FOR HEALTHCARE OUTCOMES

While I have pointed out some of the shortcomings of transparency of clinical quality measures, I am not saying that transparency is not valuable in
quality improvement efforts. For example, it has helped in reducing the mortality of cardiac surgery in New York State when such transparency became
public policy under the leadership of Mark Chassin who was state health
commissioner at that time and now leads the Joint Commission. Chassin
notes that the revelation of the hospital and surgeon-specific outcomes led to
a variety of process improvements that included replacing some surgeons,
implementing a stabilization period before surgery, and making sure the
more experienced surgeons were operating on the most difficult cases.[18]
Surgeons also were more likely to screen out and decline the most severe and
desperate cases when knowing their results would be public. This did not
appear to worsen overall cardiac outcomes, suggesting that poor operative
risks may do better without surgery. The American ethos is to do something
actively even when the risk/benefit ratio is high. This does not necessarily
make for sound clinical judgment. The mentality to "go for it on fourth
down," to use a football analogy, is often too risky.

Transparency has been particularly important concerning surgical outcomes. One reason is that surgical outcomes are very dependent on operator
skill[19] and the effectiveness of operative processes including timing of pro-
phylactic antibiotics and other items on the surgical bundle.[20] In contrast,
while primary care measures of preventive care and control of chronic conditions are also dependent on clinical processes, they also depend on factors
beyond the clinician's control such as the extent of patient activation and
medication compliance.

Makary recommends transparency of the National Practioner Databank
for patient consumers.[21] Currently only state medical boards and medical
staff credentialing offices may query the database. It is hard to disagree with
this suggestion. However, I would go further to suggest that physician credentialing and hospital privileges should be not a matter that can be subject
to tort law. While health courts have been suggested as a venue to deal with
medical liability cases,[22] I am suggesting that such courts should also have
jurisdiction on matters of physician disciplining and privileging. Recently I
was on Capitol Hill advocating for federal funding of a demonstration project

for health courts, when a democratic legislative aide inquired would such a health court help identify and discipline unsafe clinicians. I realized that it would make for a more balanced argument for healthcare courts if both medical liability and medical disciplinary actions were taken out of the civil courts and into a court with specially trained judges, lawyers (including some MD-JDs), and expert witnesses not chosen by either side. The tort system as it is currently constituted may inhibit hospitals and other clinicians from reporting problematic clinicians to state boards. Hopefully both sides of the aisle see the benefit of testing a new approach for both addressing medical liability and disciplining physicians.

ETHICAL IMPLICATIONS OF MINIMIZATION OF VARIANCE

Not every patient benefits from minimizing variance in clinical practice although the prevailing ethos is to treat medical care as just another industry where minimizing the variance is desirable. Some patients may actually be harmed by reduced variation because several patients possess "outlier" characteristics that differ significantly from those in the study population from which practice guidelines are derived. This is often the case with patients with multiple morbidities that may have led to their being excluded from the clinical studies that are used to determine the practice guidelines. Hence applying practice guidelines to such patients may not benefit them or even harm them. For example, the population of patients with diabetic renal disease appears conclusively to benefit from the use of angiotensin converting enzyme inhibitors (ACEI) from a summary of clinical studies.[23] However, other studies demonstrate that African Americans are three to four times more likely to develop angioedema, marked swelling of the lips and throat, that can result in fatal choking in some instances.[24] That information is difficult to integrate with the larger, better-known studies showing the benefits of ACEI medication. Thus guidelines may yield superior results for a largely white study population but not for this particular subpopulation not well represented in the clinical trial. However, if a physician has many African American patients in her clinical practice that are more likely to need to deviate from the standard guideline that could reflect poorly on her performance measures. These individuals would benefit from a physician's clinical judgment that *departs* from the standard approach by taking into consideration individual "outlier" characteristics. Thus one needs a physician's sound clinical judgment, which includes considering various probabilities of clinical subsets as well as the knowledge of the latest evidence to chart a safe course in the treatment of medically complex diseases. Most public policy decision-makers are not aware of this nuanced nature of medical practice or how it can impact on quality measurements. Policy makers are not master clinicians and many are not clinicians at all.

Quality medical care then differs significantly from the model of industrial quality control. Medical care requires more individualization; in contrast, statistical quality control[25] is a method of standardizing a procedure borrowed from the manufacturing industry where there is no reason for one part to deviate from the next. It is important to retain the role of the medical professional, nurse as well as physician, who is capable of independent judgment without having to devote excessive time justifying to an insurance or accrediting bureaucracy reasons for that deviation. Nurenberg, an experienced general internist, notes the difficulty and frustration today in practicing an individualized approach to patient care because of bureaucratic regulatory constraints.[26] His experience is typical as primary care and other types of physicians increasingly find a greater portion of their time is spent justifying any deviation from a standard algorithm of care to both insurers and practice managers. While the public expects their physicians to retain professional responsibility to take the particulars of their unique clinical circumstances into account rather than devolve into mere technicians of a population-based algorithm, the corporate medical managers feel otherwise as they mimic their manufacturing counterparts.

The respected philosopher Stephen Toulmin expressed concern that the healthcare insurance organization within its bureaucratic control could limit professional authority and discretion and reduce the moral autonomy of the physician.[27] The Hastings Center report on the Health Care Quality Improvement movement (HCQI)[28] notes that, in addition to concern for preserving professional integrity, the HCQI movement needs to pay attention to and respect patients' values and how they are impacted by HCQI measurements and processes. The primacy of patient autonomy is definitely being challenged by a focus on population-based healthcare standards of clinical care. With a European perspective, Norheim points out that there is a certain presumptuousness in evidence-based medicine in assuming that a patient wants the intervention simply because it has been shown to be effective for a population of patients.[29] He also observed that clinical evidence at best generates a provisional truth rather than an absolute truth until the next subsequent study modifies the preponderance of clinical evidence.

Davidoff (former editor of the *Annals of Internal Medicine*) et al. noted the clinical conundrum whereby carefully designed clinical studies seek to minimize the confounding effects of clinical context while actual clinical circumstances are inherently context dependent.[30] One must ask if there are essential limits to quality improvement that have not yet been fully explored or understood epistemologically by the purveyors of this technology.

It is instructive, I believe, to consider the postmodern concept advanced by Deleuze and Guatteri that rhizomatic policy structures, as opposed to a rigid central bureaucracy, are better for developing humane organizations.[31] The rhizome, like the roots of a tree, has a multiplicity of connections which are non-centric. The power of the root is that it is not centrally focused in one area but at the same time it is interconnected and communicates with the tree in terms of nutritive connections. The rhizome in its multiplicity avoids being "overcoded," that is over-controlled, over-simplified, and over-centralized. Primary care practice is in danger of being "overcoded" by HEDIS indicators, and PCMH downloads, while the physician is being reduced to a computerized technocrat.

It is prudent to consider some of the unintended consequences of performance measurements in the United Kingdom. Mannion and Braithwaite report they identified 20 dysfunctional consequences including measurement fixation, tunnel vision, silo development, increased inequality, overcompensation, undercompensation, gaming, bullying, and reduced staff morale among other disagreeable results.[32] Financial incentives may not be particularly conducive to proper clinical behavior. An American study found wide variation and inaccuracy of quality measures when assessing CMS criteria for "meaningful use" of the Electronic Health Record (EHR).[33] The authors note that if the accuracy of the EHR quality reports is not improved then it is unlikely such reporting can actually lead to improved quality of care. I would add to their concerns about inaccuracy that the unintended consequences of electronic measurement and reporting of quality is gaming of the system and worse. If a clinician is inaccurately and falsely accused of providing inferior clinical care, what impact does that have on her mental state and attitude to providing clinical care?

David Eddy, a founder of the quality improvement movement, observed that two types of judgments were involved in evidence-based clinical decision making, one scientific and one values based.[34] He has noted that a professional type of interaction between physician and patient is necessary for the second type of judgment.[35] I concur with his assessment and would also contend that professional judgment is frequently required for the first type of judgment as a patient's care may require a departure from the standard practice because of extenuating clinical factors as enumerated above. Some degree of physician autonomy and medical professionalism is still needed for optimal healthcare delivery although one should still expect that decision-making to be based on valid propositions, clinical evidence, and the best currently available information. This can only happen if physicians and nurses are well trained, keep up with recent studies, and are accorded some measure of professional judgment and autonomy. If not, the practice of medicine ceases to be respected as a professional endeavor and clinical quality will suffer regardless of what is being measured and by whom.

HEALTHCARE DISPARITIES

Systems that are designed to improve healthcare for the entire population may have the effect of improving it for the privileged and above-the-median income patient, but actually worsen care for the poor. If a physician cares for the sickest, most complex, least compliant, and poorest patients, then he or she will be at a disadvantage if his or her clinical *outcomes* are measured, and reported, and remuneration is based on these process measures and outcomes. Conversely, physicians treating a wealthier and healthier population with greater social supports have an advantage in outcomes. Studies have shown that patients with lower socioeconomic status have a higher readmission rate post-coronary angioplasty,[36] more adverse events after hip replacement,[37] and a higher readmission rate and higher one-year mortality for congestive heart failure.[38] While risk adjustment models for socioeconomic status have been developed from administrative databases, they do not take into consideration extenuating social factors such as family social networks, social cohesion, and social capital.[39] Moreover, most physician-specific databases such as Pay-for-Performance do not factor social items into these risk adjustments, so even as the models are developed further they may not be applied in the clinical evaluative settings where they are needed for accurate assessment of clinician performance through adjustment for confounding social factors.

Distrust in physicians is already a major concern for vulnerable minorities and their clinicians.[40] This is particularly important because distrust of physicians by their patients worsens medical compliance.[41] Revelation of their physicians' poorer outcomes when left unadjusted for sociological factors is likely to intensify distrust and poor compliance. Thus, such performance-based measures are going to exacerbate differences between the haves and the have-nots as was already observed in the English study noted above. Physicians caring for the lower socioeconomic groups may well receive lower ratings and reimbursements based on several factors beyond their control. The principles of justice and non-malfeasance will be violated when poor people, their physicians, and their patient-physician relationships are damaged by dissemination of data uncorrected for social factors.

OBJECTIVE EVIDENCE AND THE SOCIAL CONSTRUCTION OF CLINICAL PRACTICE GUIDELINES

Perhaps nowhere is postmodern thought more relevant than in the construction of clinical practice guidelines. The interpretation of medical evidence, even as clinical science progresses, is socially constructed by selected experts influenced by funding sources, other power relationships, and personal benefit. Guideline development does not emanate directly from "pure" medical evidence resulting from clinical studies; rather, it requires interpretation arising from complex intellectual and social interactions among individuals and institutions that include power relationships as well as hard data calculations.

Committee members shaping guidelines have their own biases, conscious or otherwise, connections to industry, professional organizations, pressure from department chairs, prospects of honorariums which may be sizeable, and other related factors. In a consumerist society, physicians are hardly immune from such considerations and some succumb to consumerist values more than others.

Moreover, evidence-based guidelines have a variable "shelf-life" after which they require updating. There is a lag time from when updated studies are done and the consensus panels meet and change the guidelines. Guidelines may be out of date for a period of months to sometimes a year or more. Also genuine differences of opinion exist in the interpretation of available data so different organizations and societies have competing practice guidelines at variance with one another, existing simultaneously, supported and advanced by different interpretations of the same data.

The published clinical data is sometimes misleading. Raspe observes that the false positive clinical trial with alpha type error is not uncommon in clinical reports.[42] This is the type of error made when a random variation is inaccurately attributed significance because of an error in statistical analysis or simply because of random variation. Moreover, Raspe notes that the differences between individual clinical care and clinical evaluative research are real and not totally reconcilable, a point that has been noted earlier as well.

Strict applications of standardized protocols have been shown to improve outcomes in selected medical disciplines such as the use of checklists in reducing anesthesia and surgical errors[43,44] as well as in reducing nosocomial infections.[45] Even though the checklist approach works in these instances, it does not mean it will work in all types of clinical care. The context, texture, and format of the medical profession varies considerably from surgery to medicine to psychiatry as different disciplines have different degrees of precision, human variables, and the degree to which they incorporate human values. Although the guidelines can be used as a starting point, patients desire their physicians to communicate in a professional yet personalized fashion with them and following a standardized protocol does not engender dialogue, communication, and the individualization of care with patient-derived values.

The quality improvement movement encourages computerized data collection, data downloads, and computerized comparisons to the mean regarding both process and outcome. Physicians who care for more difficult patients, either more complex or less compliant, will come out of the data

mining appearing worse than physicians who treat wealthier, more compliant, less socially complex or needy patients. Modifiers for the more complex
social factors are for the most part seriously lacking or generally underuti-
lized in the Pay-for-Performance applications. One could also foresee arguments that such modifiers are unfair and even possibly illegal. Postmodern
legal thought including critical legal studies emphasizes the relativism of law
and the hybridization of law and politics.[46] However current political correct-
ness would clearly oppose such a socioeconomic correction factors as unfairly disadvantaging the lower socioeconomic groups even though the absence
of one could have an unintended negative effect of disadvantage for those
practitioners who care for the poor.

Over a decade ago Eddy described the state of performance measurement
as "expensive, incomplete, and distorting."[47] The issues he noted were the
probabilistic nature of outcomes, low frequency of many outcomes, long
delays before an effect occurred, and only modest control by the physician on
outcomes, among others. Although these shortcomings have not yet been
overcome, various healthcare stakeholders are urging computerized performance measurement implementation before the impact of such a policy has
been fully evaluated.

A recent example of the rush to implement practice guidelines before the
clinical science has been fully evaluated is the guideline recommendations by
the Joint Commission and the Institute for Health Improvement (IHI), two
respected and important organizations, to recommend normalization of the
blood glucose in the intensive care setting. Perhaps in keeping with the
American ethos that more must be better, they developed these guidelines
with limited studies supporting them. Subsequent studies showed higher, not
lower, mortality with very tight glucose control.[48,49] IHI promptly revised
their recommendations and noted the ambiguity after this study was published[50] but thousands of hospitals were already busy adopting tight control
with at best ambivalent clinical results. Groopman and Hartzband noted that
the hospitals and physicians came under intensive pressure to conform to the
Joint Commission guidelines or face a lowering of their public ratings.[51] The
power exerted by such organizations and the published online ratings are
very substantial and their bureaucratic approach is going to impact how the
medical profession and medical professionals view themselves and their own
agency.

Deleuze and Guattari speak of a "cybernetic servitude" in a control society under late capitalism.[52] That sounds eerily like the current state of medical practice in the twenty-first century.

Surveys[53] evaluating physician burnout in the United States identified the
leading causes to include performing too many bureaucratic tasks, feeling
like a cog the in medical industry, and increasing computerization of medical

practice.[54] A dissatisfied, harried professional is hardly a guarantee of excellent quality outcomes.

An understanding of the human limits of knowledge is an essential prerequisite to having an informed public policy. Foucault's observations about the interdependency of knowledge and the power structure in the clinical and academic settings are relevant in this regard. "Knowledge does not 'reflect' power relations; . . . it is immanent in them."[55] Power is an essential element to giving voice to best practices, often determined by national organizations with their own power structures and private as well as public agendas. Even as objectivity is a desired goal, a degree of subjectivity is inevitable in medical practice and the development of practice guidelines. Bureaucrats and corporations apparently wish to implement a control model that copies the manufacturing and service industries. However, the loss of professionalism in medical practice will have undesirable consequences that are inherent in such a centralized bureaucratic control model of care delivery.

Hardt and Negri note that technoculture in postmodernity emphasizes "imbrications of space, capital, and networked computers."[56] The consolidation of healthcare systems and health insurance into complex, integrated healthcare systems follows a similar pattern of overlapping layers of capital, medical expertise, corporate communicative hegemony, and networked computers. Such concentration of power will influence what constitutes medical knowledge and will likely diminish the humanist elements in medical practice. Moreover the aforementioned example shows that it has the power to compel physicians to adopt clinical practices before they are fully vetted and verified. The hubris of the power elite applies in medical practice as well as other fields and disciplines.

CONCLUSIONS

Caution is recommended before computerized measurement of physician performance is widely adopted and embraced. The benefits of Pay-for-Performance and other physician-specific reports should be substantiated before wide-scale implementation occurs. This requires carefully designed studies to detect unintended consequences several of which have already come to light in the United States and the United Kingdom. Healthcare organizations must be careful not to lower standards of *process* for patients in the lower socioeconomic groups but care should be taken not to disadvantage the physicians who provide healthcare to those patients where outcomes are often less than for those in higher socioeconomic circumstances. The need exists for research appropriate risk modifiers for patient population characteristics based on socioeconomic factors and to use them appropriately in such analyses. The development and maintenance of databases robust enough to take these modifying factors into consideration is not a standard practice today by agencies in the quality measurement business but should be essential before implementing physician outcomes performance and reimbursement on a widespread basis.

New health policies should be thoroughly evaluated in a controlled fashion before wide-scale implementation. Expert consensus panels would hopefully not consider changing a clinical care practice without such a thorough evaluation process and sufficient supporting data, and that degree of caution should be exercised with important health policies on healthcare delivery as well as clinical care.

Patients benefit from the preservation of the individual physician's professionalism as well as that of other healthcare professionals. This requires preserving the role of their independent judgment in taking into consideration the best available evidence and the patient's unique characteristics. Certain dimensions of quality in healthcare delivery will require an active role for supervisory clinical leaders as well as documentation of performance data. The evidence base of medical practice is ever changing, influenced by scientific progress, power relationships and other human factors. Humility concerning the limits of human knowledge should also inform public policy concerning healthcare. Judicious progress in healthcare delivery has been made with quality improvement initiatives and will continue but caution must be exercised not to diminish medical or nursing professionalism and its benefits in a mass of bureaucratic control and electronic data downloads. This will require more ethical and sociological inquiry as well as outcomes and comparative effectiveness studies to fully understand these important issues. Care must be taken to avoid a rigid central bureaucracy that layers capital, clinical expertise, and networked computer data downloads. There is a need to maintain the energy and dynamism of a rhizomatically creative and somewhat independent medical profession. New methods of disciplinary actions for clinicians should include consideration of health courts with specific expertise in such matters.

We must learn not only "what works best" but also to understand the limits of the types of knowledge developed in the computer age as well as how to preserve an older type of knowledge that clinical judgment and medical professionalism embodies so that patients can benefit from both types of knowledge and wisdom. We need humility of organizations as well as individuals to understand cautiously that there are limits to human knowledge, including medical knowledge. To ignore the reality of such limits imperils rather than improves human healthcare.

NOTES

1. Kass L.http://www.brainyquote.com/quotes/quotes/l/leonkass.282439.html

2. Foucault M. *Discipline and Punish: The Birth of the Prison.* Gallimard, 1975.

3. Chassin M., Hannan E. L., DeBuono B. A. Benefits and hazards of reporting medical outcomes publicly. *N J Engl Med*, 1996; 334:394–398.

4. Kiele C. I., Alison J. J., Williams O. D., Person S. D., Waver M. T., Weisssman N. W. Improving Quality Improvement using achievable benchmarks for physician feedback. *JAMA* 2001; 285:2871–2879.

5. Peterson L. A., Woodard L. D., Urecht T., Daw C., Sookanan S. Does pay-for-performance improve the quality of care? *Ann Intern Med* 2006; 145:265–272.

6. Li B. L., Brown W. A., Ampil F. L. Patient Compliance is Critical for Equivalent Outcomes for Breast Cancer. *Ann Surg.* 2000 June, 231(6): 883–889.

7. Casalino L. The unintended consequences of measuring quality on the quality of medical care. *NEJM.* 341:1147–1150, 1999.

8. Thygeson M., Morrisey L., Ulstad V. Adaptive leadership and the practice of medicine: complexity-based approach to reframing the doctor-patient relationship. *J. Eval. Clin Practice* 16:1009–15, 2010.

9. Peterson L. A., Woodard L. D., Urecht T., Daw C., Sookanan S. Does pay-for-performance improve the quality of care? *Ann Intern Med* 2006; 145:265–27.

10. No Shot No Doc: Pediatricians refuse unvaccinated children http://today.msnbc.msn.com/id/44356327/ns/today-today_health/t/no-shot-no-doc-pediatricians-refuse-unvaccinated-kids/.

11. Godzich W. *Afterword the Postmodern Explained J-F Lyotard.* Univ Minnesota. 1992, p. 114.

12. HEDIS Indicators. http://www.ncqa.org/tabid/1415/Default.aspx. Accessed September 18, 2012.

13. Adams J. L., Mehrotra A., Thomas J. W., McGlynn E. A. Physician Cost Profiling—Reliability and Risk of Misclassification. *N Engl J Med.* 2010, 362:1014–1021.

14. Woodhandler S., Himmelstein D. Why pay for performance may be incompatible with quality improvement. *BMJ* 2012, 345: e5015.

15. The Joint Commission: Ongoing Professional Practice. http://www.jointcommission.org/AccreditationPrograms/CriticalAccessHospitals/Standards/09_FAQs/MS/Ongoing_Professional_Practice_Evaluation.htm.

16. Uncertainty principle Wikipedia. http://en.wikipedia.org/wiki/Uncertainty_principle

17. Urban Institute. Patient Centered Medical Home Recognition Tools. 412338-patient-centered-medical-home-rec-tools.pdf

18. Chassin M. R. Achieving and maintaining improved quality: lessons from New York State and cardiac surgery. *Health Aff.* 21(4): 40–51, 2002.

19. Twijnstra A. R., Blikkenddall M. D., van Zwet E. W., et al. Predictors of successful surgical outcome in laparoscopic hysterectomy. *Obstet Gynecol.* 119(4): 700–708, 2012.

20. "SCIP"ping antibiotic prophylaxis guidelines in trauma. Smith B. P., Fox N., Fakhro A., et al. *J Trauma Acute Care Surg* 73(2): 452–456, 2012.

21. Makary M. *Unaccountable: What Hospitals Won't Tell You and How Transparency Can Revolutionize Health Care.* New York: Bloomsbury: 2012 and Newsweek September 24, 2012, 46–36.

22. Tobias C. W. Healthcare Courts: Panacea or Palliative? *Univ Richmond Law Review.* 40:49–52, 2005.

23. Kshirsagar A. V., Joy M. S., Hogan S. L., et al. Effects of ACE inhibitors in diabetic and nondiabetic renal disease. *Am J Kidney Dis.* 2000; 35(4): 695–707.

24. Brown N. J., Ray W. A., Snowden M., et al. Black Americans have an increased incidence of Angiotensin converting enzyme inhibitor. *Clin Pharm Therapeutics.* 60:8–13,1996.

25. Statistical Qualtiy Control Weily. http://www.wiley.com/college/sc/reid/chap6.pdf. Accessed April 27, 2013.

26. Norenberg D. D. The demise of primary care: a diatribe from the trenches. *Ann Intern Med* 2009; 150:725–726.

27. Toulmin S. E. Medical institutions and their moral constraints, in E. Bulger, Reiser S. J., ed. *Integrity in Healthcare Institutions.* Iowa City: University of Iowa Press, 1990.

28. Jennings B., Baily M. A., Bottrell M., Lynn J., eds. Heath Care Quality Improvement: Ethical and Regulatory Issues. http://www.thehastingscenter.org/Publications/SpecialReports/Detail.aspx?id=1342.

29. Norheim O. F. The role of formal outcome evaluations in health policy making: a normative approach. *Evidence-based Practice in Medicine and Healthcare.* Eds., Meulen R. T., Biller-Andorno N., Lenk, C., Lie R. Berlin: Springer Verlag, 2005, Chap 15.

30. Davidoff F., Batalden P., Stevens D., Ogrinic G., Mooney S. Publication guidelines for improvement studies in healthcare: evolution of the SQUIRE project. *Ann Intern Med.* 2008; 149:670–676.

31. Deleuze G., Guattari F. *A Thousand Plateaus.* Minneapolis: University of Minnesota Press. Trans. Massoni B. 1987.

32. Mannion R., Braithwaite J. Unintended consequences of performance measurement in healthcare: 20 salutary lessions form the English National Health Service. *Internal Medicine Journal.* 42(5):569–574, 2012.

33. Kern K. M., Malhotra S., Barron Y., et al. Accuracy of Electronically Reported "Meaningful Use" Clinical Quality Measures. *Ann Int Med* 158:77–83, 2013.

34. Eddy D. M. Clinical Decision Making: From theory into practice-anatomy of a decision. *JAMA* 1990; 263(3):441–443.

35. Tunis S. R. Reflections on science, judgment, and value in evidence-based decision making: a conversation with David Eddy. *Health Affairs* 2007; 26(4): w500–w515.

36. Denvir M. A., Lee A. J., Rysdale J., Walker A., Eteiba H., Starkey R., Pell J. P. Influence of socioeconomic status on clinical outcomes and quality of life after percutaneous coronary intervention. *J Epi Comm Health* 2006; 60:1085–1088.

37. Agabitti N., Piciotto S., Ceronini G., et al. The influence of socioeconomic status on utilization and outcomes of elective hip replacement. *International J Qual Health Care* 2007; 19(1):37–44.

38. Rathore S., Masoudi F. A., Yongfei Wang, Curtis J. Socioeconomic status, treatment and outcomes among elderly patients hospitalized with heart failure. *Am Heart J* 2006; 152: 371–378.

39. Rosen A. K., Reid R., Broeremling A. M., Rakovski C. C. Applying a risk-adjustment framework to primary care: can we improve on existing measures? *Ann Fam Med* 2003; 1: 41–44.

40. Armstrong K., Ravell K. L., McMurphy S. Race/ethnic differences in physician distrust in America. http://www.medscape.com/viewarticle/561477_4. Accessed July 25, 2009.

41. Kerse N., Buelow S., Mainous A. G., Young G., Coster G., Arroll B. Patient-physician relationship and medication compliance. *Annals of Fam Med* 2: 455–461, 2004.

42. H. Raspe. Clinical evaluative research: which patient benefit, how and when? A contribution to a European discussion. Ch 12 in *Evidenced-based Practice in Medicine and Healthcare.* Eds. Meulen R. T., Biller-Andorno N., Lenk, C., Lie R. Berlin: Springer Verlag 2005.

43. March M. G., Crowley J. J. An evaluation of anesthesiologists' present checkout method: the validity of the FDA checklist. *Anesthesiology.* 1991; 75: 724–729.

44. Haynes A. B., Weiser T. G., Berry W. R., et al. A surgical safety checklist to reduce morbidity and mortality in a global population. *N Engl J Med.* 2009; 360:491–499.

45. Wachter R., Provonost P. The hundred thousand lives campaign. A scientific and policy review. *Joint Commission J Qual Safety* 2006; 26(11):621–627.

46. Fruehwald S. The Emperor has no Clothes: Postmodern legal thought and cognitive science. *Georgia S. U. Law Review* 23(3): 374–424.

47. Eddy D. M. Performance Measurement: Problems and Solutions. *Health Affairs* 1998; 17(4): 7–25.

48. The NICE-SUGAR Study Investigators. Intensive versus conventional glucose control in critically ill patients. *N Engl J Med* 360: 1283–97, 2009.

49. Kavanagh B. P. Glucose in the ICU-Evidence, Guidelines and Outcomes. *N Engl J Med* 367(13): 1259–60, 2012.

50. http://www.ihi.org/knowledge/Pages/Changes/ImplementEffectiveGlucoseControl.aspx. Accessed September 27, 2012.

51. Groopman J., Hartzband P. Why Quality of Care is Dangerous. *Wall Street Journal* April 8, 2009. Opinion.

52. Deleuze Giles, Guattari Felix. *Capitalism and Schizphrenia*. Minneapolis: Univ Minnesota, 1987, and *From Schizophrenia to Social Control*. Holland E. W. In Deleuze and Guattari, *New Mappings in Politics, Philosophy, and Culture*, University of Minnesota 1998, pp. 65–72.

53. Shanafelt T. D., Boone S., Tan L., et al. Burnout and satisfaction with work-life balance among US physicians relative to the US population. *Arch Intern Med* 172:1377–1385, 2012.

54. Peckham C. Burnout Severity and its Effect on Physicians. *Medscape*. http://www. medscape.com/viewarticle/781161_2. Accessed March 31, 2013.

55. Sheridan A. *Michel Foucault: The Will to Truth*. Tavistock, London, 1980, p. 220.

56. Dean J. in *Empire's New Clothes*. Ed. Passavant P. A., Dean J. New York: Routledge, 2004, The Networked Empire.

Chapter Five

The Uneven Encounter between Postmodern Expectations and Corporate Control of Medical Practice

". . . the corporate system does not offer incremental reforms to the framework of professional dominance in medicine but has swept it away completely. . ." —James C. Robinson *The Corporate Practice of Medicine*[1]

"Questioning the ostensibly unquestionable premises of our way of life is arguably the most urgent of services we owe our fellow humans and ourselves." —Zygmunt Bauman[2]

CORPORATIONS IN ASCENDANCY: DO CORPORATIONS PRACTICE MEDICINE?

Game, Set, Match, Championship, so to speak, Professor Robinson ends his book, *The Corporate Practice of Medicine*[3] by trumpeting the triumph of corporate medicine over the individual practioner model of medical practice dominated by physicians that persisted through much of the twentieth century. It is hard to refute the dominance of corporations over medical professionals in the twenty-first century. Many physicians still may try to resist, but they will find it economically difficult to do so. It will become even more difficult in the coming era of Accountable Care Organizations (ACOs). ACOs require a greater degree of coordination and capital investment both for computerized systems and in assuming risk for costs of care that are considerably more than an individual practioner or even groups of practitioners can provide. The ACOs under development by CMS and provider organizations would assume responsibility and risk for at least 5,000 Medicare patients for three years,[4] and so the provider organization is assuming the insurance risk itself.

Corporations beginning in the 1970s recognized the profitability of medical care and formed the nucleus of this industry. Companies involved in hospital care, integrated healthcare delivery systems, specialized care such as nursing homes, long term-acute care, rehabilitation, dialysis services, cardiology services, mental health services, medical billing and management services, and many other aspects of medical care have grown enormously. These provider organizations now compete for supremacy while the highly influential insurers do likewise. Business professors like Robinson have faith in market forces to produce value; Robinson sees the corporate system of healthcare as superior to the prior model of professional dominance.[5] At the same time, Robinson warns of some dangers, "Through its economic dynamism, the corporate system seems to undermine the social and political basis of its own support."[6] This is a strong claim that economic dynamism, much admired in corporate circles, corrodes its social and political support. This suggests that economic success can undermine the social fabric. The economist Jeffrey Sachs observes that efficiency is only one important goal of an economy and that fairness and sustainability are important economic considerations that globalized corporations are less able to provide.[7] In healthcare, access for the socially and economically disadvantaged is an important bioethical principle and the driving force behind the Obama administration's Patient Protection and Affordable Care Act.[8] Discussion over this principle dominated much of the political debate in the 2012 presidential election. Sustainability must also be considered not only in terms of the global environment but with regard to the human ecology of medical practice. In this regard both sides of the political spectrum view a corporate bureaucratic approach as the only option, though one view is more privatized and the other more public. Daniel Bell observed in his book, *The Cultural Contradictions of Capitalism,* that a secularized hedonistic culture was favorable to the corporate mass marketing of consumer goods.[9] It raises the issue that corporate successes in controlling the provision of healthcare may have untoward effects on the social aspects of healthcare delivery as well as on total costs.

Surprisingly, corporations are legally and explicitly prohibited from practicing medicine. In Alabama, for example, an attorney general opinion appears to allow a corporation to employ a physician to provide medical services if the corporation does not interfere with the physician's independent medical judgment.[10]

> "The state does not prohibit a physician from working for a corporation as long as the corporation does not exercise control over the physician's independent medical judgment." In New York state: "The use of the word 'person' in the physician licensing statute means that a corporation may not practice medi-

cine. Corporations may not employ licensed professionals to practice medicine." See *People v. John H. Woodbury Dermatological Inst.*, 85 N.E. 697 (N.Y. 1908).

In Pennsylvania:

A court held that a licensed practitioner may not practice among the public as a servant of an unlicensed person or a Corporation. See *Neill v. Gimbel Bros., Inc.*, 199 A. 178, 182 (Pa. 1938).

But: "A health care practitioner may practice the healing arts as an employee or independent contractor of a health care facility or health care provider or an affiliate of a health care facility or health care provider established to provide health care." See 35 P.S. § 448.817a (2006).

And the Tennessee law is one of the most explicit:

"The practice of medicine by non-professional corporations is allowed if the employment relationship between the physician and the corporation is evidenced by a written contract with a job description and with language that does not restrict the physician from *exercising independent medical judgment* in diagnosing and treating patients. If so, then the corporation shall not be deemed to be engaged in the practice of medicine." See Tenn. Code Ann. § 63-6-204(c) 2006.

So legislators, both in the past and more recently, have believed it necessary to make sure that corporations not dictate diagnosis and treatment to physicians. Have these laws succeeded in doing what they were intended to do? Healthcare corporations may implement practice guidelines, order sets, and recommended protocols but must leave some discretion to physicians or so the laws seem to indicate.

However, there are two well known admission guidelines, Milliman[11] guidelines and InterQual[12] guidelines, developed as proprietary actuarial products, and used by health insurers to determine whether or not to pay for hospital admissions.

Milliman Inc. describes their product as follows: "Milliman Care Guidelines® are annually updated, evidence-based clinical guidelines that span the continuum of care, including chronic care and behavioral health management. Providing much more than authorization criteria, they drive high-quality care through such tools as care pathway tables, flagged quality measures, and integrated medical evidence."[13] McKesson, Interqual's owner states, "InterQual Criteria cover the medical and behavioral health continuums of care. InterQual products are widely used by hospitals and payers because they understand that the rigor used to develop the criteria helps to ensure quality—the right care at the right time in the right setting."[14] The InterQual

Criteria are used by over 300 health plans, 4,000 hospitals, and the Centers for Medicare & Medicaid Services (CMS). It is a very successful product and plays a significant role in determining how and when patients are admitted to hospitals. One InterQual employee wrote an article extolling its virtues and philosophy, "over the years, the InterQual team worked hard, constantly improving and updating the criteria."[15] That may or may not be so, but one also needs to ask what social as well as medical impacts on healthcare do such products and their prominence have on the medical professions.

These actuarial products are designed to be used to set criteria for payments to hospitals and physicians for inpatient care. A critical view of their impact emerges from the description in *Critical Condition: How Health Care in America Became Big Business & Bad Medicine* by Donald L. Barlett and James B. Steele,[16] journalists who have won two Pulitzer prizes. Milliman guidelines, they observed, brought the so-called "drive through deliveries," setting the best-case scenarios for hospital length of stay as the *standard* for length of stays and associated payments. They also note that Milliman indicates that their guidelines are only tools in medical decision-making and not the decision itself. But when payers base payment decisions on these guidelines they become significantly more than that. Hospitals need to be paid for the services they render so when the payer uses actuarial guidelines to determine payment to the hospital, its staff needs to heed those guidelines if they want to remain in business.

So the actuarial guidelines marketed as products by corporations interconnect to the commercial practices of insurance companies (or federal contractors providing government sponsored medical insurance services) and these in turn interconnect to the corporate hospital/healthcare delivery system. Together these interconnections create a corporate nexus that comes close to simulating the corporate practice of medicine while still retaining the role of clinicians, albeit in a diminished way. Each component is legal, since actual medical orders are written by clinicians, and even standardized order sets must at least be signed by an individual medical professional, who may be a licensed nurse practitioner or physician assistant as well as a physician. But the individual medical professional now operates in the framework of substantial corporate control.

Most if not all evidence-based guidelines contain some value judgments. Clinical evidence does not directly imply a specific guideline without value judgments being used to make the guidelines. Eddy, an expert in quality improvement, noted that the ethical assessment of an evidence-based guideline is often entwined with its economic cost analysis.[17] The value judgment implicit in these guidelines often comes in the form of a criterion that the shorter the stay the better the medical care or, at least, the better the medical care "value." Barlett and Steele note that both the American College of Obstetricians and Gynecologists and the American Society of Pediatrics objected to a 24-hour stay for vaginal deliveries that was the duration approved by the Milliman guideline.[18] The strong reaction that this guideline evoked from physicians and patients led to the federal legislation known as the Mothers and Newborn Health Protection Act of 1996[19] It mandated that health insurers pay for at least 48 hours for a vaginal delivery and 96 hours for a delivery requiring a caesarean section (surgical excision) and prohibited the insurer from requiring authorization for a stay of those lengths. A clinical study demonstrated that a short length of stay increases the risk of readmission for women who had a caesarean section.[20]

In another publication evaluating effect of hospitalization length on clinical outcomes, investigators using the National Trauma Data Bank found that those patients who followed guidelines for length of stay had higher mortality.[21] Rutledge, using a statewide database, found that the Milliman and Robertson guidelines for surgery were at wide variance from patients' actual length of stay and noted that applying them could hurt some patients.[22] There is a notable lack of further studies of how actuarial guidelines for admission have impacted the quality of healthcare outcomes. It would hardly be surprising, if economic values predominate in actuarial products.

Many practice guidelines may value best clinical outcomes, but actuarial companies lean toward a greater interest in efficiency with regard to costs of care since their purpose is to help moderate expenditures. The actuarial companies note they are merely providing guidelines, they do not compel the payers to use them, and the payers do not compel the physicians or hospital to get paid. But economic reality does make the guidelines important to hospitals and the clinicians that work in them.

Milliman was sued by Dr. Thomas Cleary and three other physicians for erroneously listing them as contributors to the Milliman pediatric guidelines, and their attributions were removed in subsequent additions of their guidelines.[23] If Milliman's contributor list was inaccurate, could other aspects of the guidelines also be inaccurate? There is certainly a need to assess the impact of any guidelines that affect clinical care. A recent study, however, found that hospitals that spent more per patient for six common diagnoses had lower inpatient mortality.[24] So quite possibly, more cost effective care may not equate to the best quality of care. Guidelines that help reduce hospital utilization may not be as value neutral as they are purported to be with regard to the clinical value of medical care. Why has this aspect not been studied in more detail? Maybe the web of corporate influence could account for the dearth of studies.

SYSTEMS THINKING IS NOT NECESSARILY LINEAR AND DETERMINISTIC

Complexity science and systems thinking suggest that recursive feedback loops, non-linear stochastic changes within a system, and emergent, hierarchal properties drive a system to value and quality improvement or conceivably toward the opposite.[25] Rather than embracing a reductionistic, controlled domain, complexity science acknowledges provinces of perplexing, counter-intuitive co-evolutionary change outside of a command and control system. According to systems theory, a healthcare system, like any system, is a dynamic complex of interrelated subsystems in a state of equilibrium created by feedback loops of information and control.[26] Its quality of care is an emergent property of the whole including the personal values, attitudes, and sensibilities of its leaders, managers, and workers. Lyotard, who often wrote in the language of systems thinking, stated "It is only in late capitalism that this hierarchal articulation has been broken and that the subsystems of technical activity have become autonomous in relation to the world of interaction."[27] For the business of medicine, the computerization of medical information has drawn attention away from the non-reductionistic, holistic aspects of medical practice into a vortex of digitized billing, computerized order entry, and a more centralized control of decision support. So while systems thinking is in fact often non-hierarchal, supporting counter-intuitive control mechanisms, the enlargement of the role of corporations in medical practice has not fully embraced systems thinking; rather, it has implemented systems of command and control. At their best corporations encourage and act upon visionary thinking as appears to have been the case with the Apple Corporation under Steven Jobs.[28] However, in my estimation, this is not the type of thinking that is being encouraged in the large corporations of the medical industry today. The use of the classical industrial model of central control has been stultifying for some healthcare organizations.

BUSINESS ETHICS: ASYMMETRIES IN THE POSTMODERN ERA

A decade ago, Eiser, Gould, and Suchman stated, "Business ethics is not an oxymoron but its grasp is tenuous because of the primacy of economic interest in the marketplace and the decline of public consensus on socially acceptable norms of conduct."[29] Since then the marginality of business ethics has been accentuated by the numerous instances of corporate malfeasance such as Enron,[30] billion dollar fines to pharmaceutical companies,[31] and the financial institution meltdown of 2008. The Sarbanes-Oxley law of 2002 was designed to make corporate boards and external auditors provide more oversight of institutions and reveal more information to shareholders, but the law has not had the impact one might have expected.[32] Republican candidates for president even called for its repeal as well as repealing other regulatory measures.[33]

More than two decades ago Robert Jackall in *Moral Mazes* describes the amoral world of the corporate manager. Through a series of over 140 interviews of corporate managers he found a practical ethos that turned personal responsibility into adroitness at public relations, the quest for advantage vanquished moral deontological considerations.[34] Nothing more recent suggests any change in this regard.

The decline of cultural norms is important in the asymmetries of postmodern life. Jameson notes the following regarding the postmodern condition: "depthlessness or the waning of moral consensus or sensibility, weakness of historicity, the rising influence of technology, and the mutation of both the objective and subjective world."[35] Corporations and the individuals that run them in healthcare and other industries do not feel the restraint of community values, historic connection, personal connection to patients, or subscription to shared moral values across communities. The business practice of "rescission" or dropping patients once they are diagnosed with serious illness is considered a sound business practice by those executives who practice it. After all, the executives can avoid facing a direct connection, personal or societal, to the sick person who is a cipher in a computer database, a faceless number after all in a distant location, an expense item in a computerized report.

Consider the following report of such business practices: "The hearing on the controversial action known as rescission, which has left thousands of Americans burdened with costly medical bills despite paying insurance premiums, began a day after President Obama outlined his proposals for revamping the nation's healthcare system. An investigation by the House Subcommittee on Oversight and Investigations showed that health insurers WellPoint Inc., UnitedHealth Group, and Assurant Inc. canceled the coverage of more than 20,000 people for technical errors in their applications, allowing the companies to avoid paying more than $300 million in medical claims over a five-year period."[36]

As long as customers (patients) are faceless numbers in an anonymous system and that is likely to remain the case, "good" business decisions can be viewed in isolation from the human toll that they might take. Postmodern ethos in general favors a type of "digitized haze" of electronic data, electronic entertainment, and "liquid" social consumerist values. Bauman[37] also points out that corporations in postmodern times exert control by uncertainty and annexation of culture through advertising, ubiquitous media presence that attenuates a sense of common purpose in the interest of private profits and the creation of a "market-led society of consumers."

If at one time a Foucauldian postmodern critique seemed to promise new ideas and expand the possible, the sheer weight of consumerist capitalism has shifted the trajectory of postmodern culture in the direction of diminished creativity and morality by dissolving the focus on future consequences in favor of the immediate experience of hyper-real pleasures of consumption. With such a focus, the act of cutting off someone's health insurance at a time when it is needed most is not only possible but viewed as a sound business practice. Max Weber nearly a century ago observed that bureaucratization, be it in government or industry, suppresses an essential part of our humanity.[38] The rescission of sick people by insurance companies and the dire consequences that may have for them appears to be a good example of such dehumanization at work in a large remote insurance bureaucracy.

FREEMAN AND STAKEHOLDER THEORY OF BUSINESS

My co-authors and I ended our article on the interface of business ethics and bioethics a decade ago on an excessively optimistic note: "The challenges to ethically based medical practice are substantial, but many interested parties working collaboratively can create the needed solutions."[39] This misplaced optimism arose from my misreading of Freeman's Stakeholder Theory of the Modern Corporation.[40] Freeman's theory held that the corporation and its management needed to be responsive to not only shareholders and customers, but also to the local community, employees, and suppliers. It implied that a normative core existed through which a dialogue among the stakeholders was engendered. Freeman ultimately based his theory on a Rawlserian appeal to distributive justice,[41] a position that clearly does not have much currency in the business world. Humans are by nature as fractious as they are cooperative, so stakeholder theory goes only so far in a thinly supported moral framework of common good in the postmodern corporation. Clearly some stakeholders have much more power and influence than others, so the influence of community stakeholders' interests now seems rather illusory. Moreover, Frederick astutely noted that a powerful cultural value in the modern corporation is "power aggrandizement," which includes the tendency toward mergers and acquisitions to expand market share and he notes that the addictive "high" that aggrandizing power produces is a defining trait of the corporate personality.[42]

Researchers surveyed a large sample of physicians who interacted with managed health insurance plans. They found that for-profit, multi-state insurance companies were the least trustworthy, followed by not-for-profit multi-state companies.[43] The most trustworthy to physicians and patients were locally controlled not-for-profits. However, such plans have become increasingly scarce as they could not accumulate sufficient capital to remain competitive. However, researchers found when not-for-profits had more than thirty percent of the market share, their trustworthiness diminished as well. Clearly size of the company, the locus of decision-making and for-profit status influence trustworthiness of an enterprise in the view of clinicians.

Thus power aggrandizement, as measured in this study of multi-state operations, for-profit status, and large market share eroded trustworthiness of the insurance companies. A large for-profit corporation whose headquarters are remote to its facilities has no ties to the local community so that vital stakeholder connections and needs are attenuated. Power aggrandizement is also influenced by the values of the corporate leadership, but in a for-profit company as well as large not-for-profit company the leaders are often in-centivized by large bonuses and promotions to meet company-designated objectives. Under such conditions, the "stakeholders" in Freeman's theory devolve to the executive, his/her boss, and their targeted economic objectives and resultant bonuses. Many stakeholders around the table count little, if at all.

BAUMAN, FOUCAULT, AND POSTMODERN BUSINESS ETHICS

In postmodern life, morality is diluted by the weakening of social norms as the diversity of norms has multiplied. Postmodernism is also oriented toward questions of relation and relativeness, both in style and substance, rather than universal underlying verifiable principles. Pulkkinen notes postmodern thinking attributes to human subjectivity such influences as power, desire, and difference.[44] Thus central questions remain of how much consensual dialogue can still occur and how much of human organization is relativistic pastiche thrown together in a cauldron where economic influences predomi-nate. Bauman challenges modernism for its equating truth with science or more specifically the corporate implementation of science in the technology of the consumerist society.[45] He asks how does one re-install ethics into the power aggrandizing world of corporations. In this regard he turns to a me-thodological individualism that relies heavily on Levinas' asymmetrical face-to-face encounter with the Other.[46] Bauman wants to liberate the self from the iron cage of bureaucracy to let the self encounter the Other and exercise moral intuition. However, he doesn't yet answer the question of how to accomplish encounters with the Other in the postmodern corporation. Kele-men and Peltonen call attention to the need to refocus a dialogue on the ethics of managing not in deontological or utilitarian mode but in a pragmat-ic, applied mode of what ethical business agency looks like in the twenty-first century.[47] Clearly it was easier to discuss ethics when there was a greater consensus on what constitutes the good, but in postmodern times we would benefit from more extensive public conversation on what form ethical business practice should and can take. There are some attempts in this regard such as Donaldson's and Dunfee's Integral Social Contracts Theory[48] but little impact of this approach is visible today. Has postmodern culture so altered the ethical terrain of the twenty-first century that social contracts have lost their hold on managers as well as professionals including physicians? Business leaders and physicians alike spend their first two formative decades of life as neither business leaders nor physicians. The environment they grow up in is very much imbued with cultural values largely derived from entertainment media, advertising media, news media, and even video games and electronic social media. The business literature notes that organizational dishonesty is harmful to corporations in many ways including degradation of reputation, loss of employees, loss of customers, loss of shareholder value, and increased employee and management stress.[49] But roots of dishonesty begin much earlier in the now commonplace academic dishonesty found in business, law, and medical students. Several interesting observations emerge from a study of academic dishonesty of marketing students in the United States and China.[50] American students who are tolerant, detached, relativistic, non-religious (in other words postmodern) are more likely to find academic dishonesty more acceptable. The strongest factor favoring dishonesty was a high score on opportunism. The Chinese students were more detached, less religious, more relativistic, and more likely to engage in dishonest academic behavior, although rates were high in both groups. Similarly in a study of business students in Eastern Europe, Central Asia, and the United States, rates of cheating ranged from fifty percent to ninety percent although more Americans were likely to indicate that cheating is ethically wrong.[51] Thus postmodern moral values appear to be ubiquitous in countries across the globe. Moreover, they are damaging to academic honesty and ultimately business ethics as well as medical professional ethics. For example, Medicare fraud is perpetuated by many different types of professionals including businessmen, physicians, and pharmacists.

THE POSTMODERN CORPORATION AND THE BIOCULTURAL MODEL

To the observations about the corporate takeover of the medical industry, one needs to add some of the unique features of medical practice that distinguish it from the other services within the economy. Getting one's medical needs attended to is not like buying a pair of shoes. It is both a "high stakes" and deeply personal service. It requires divulging personal information, hopefully developing a trusting clinical relationship, receiving reliable, evidence-based diagnosis and treatment that are not based on the physicians' or the corporations' financial interest but on the patient's personal interests. It also requires the application of medical expertise in a very personalized fashion as disease has highly variable manifestations in different individuals that include biological, psychological, social, ethnic, and cultural differences. This distinguishes the medical industry from other industries such as the airline industry. All of these aspects have become further diversified and complex in postmodern times. Morris places emphasis on the interplay between culture and illness, and calls for a bio-cultural model that examines the narratives and micro-ethics of individual patients.[52] He notes that the postmodern vision of healthcare does not hold many answers because it is very cognizant of contingency on unknown or uncontrollable dimensions. He chooses to view this optimistically but I would caution that simply following our current course will not create a rosy outlook for a bio-cultural sensitive perspective. By turning the medical industry over to the large for-profit and not-for-profit corporations, a 2.7 trillion dollar technology-driven industry has emerged without much concern for individual narratives. Many patients, physicians, nurses, legislators, and taxpayers are dismayed with the many non-linear feedback loops of the medical industrial complex but technologically costly feedback loops not patient-centered or even health-centered ones. At times American medicine is extraordinary effective, frequently extravagant, often wasteful, and sometimes dangerous. The corporate takeover that Professor Robinson described is accurate but flawed in its inception and outcome, if a responsive and efficient system is desired. The nature of healthcare inhibits it from acting like a free commodity market. Most healthcare markets tend to become dominated by a few insurers that have a large market share, and often are very large, multi-state, publicly-traded private bureaucracies. The U.S. Government Accountability Office (GAO) found that the median share of the largest healthcare insurance carrier in a region was forty-seven percent, and in sixteen markets the largest carrier had a fifty percent share or higher.[53] This hardly makes for a competitive market in healthcare insurance. The delivery systems are soon to follow this trend of merger and conglomeration and private practice will become scarce in the future in the era of Accountable Care Organizations that will need to spread the risk of care over a large population of patients. The postmodern corporation has made substantial inroads into the realm of medical practice leaving the landscape of medical practice forever altered but certainly not necessarily cost effective or culturally and personally sensitive in its delivery of care.

The characteristics of the postmodern corporation support a very "thin" notion of business ethics. For example a Commonwealth Fund report recently noted that for-profit Medicaid managed care plan are both more costly and have lower indicators of quality care[54] than not-for-profit. Clearly the myth of the superiority of the free market as a means to cost effective, high quality care has been exposed. The uncertainty of "liquid modern" values in a moral relativist environment weakens the patient-provider relationship especially when controlled by a remote executive uninhibited by the Hippocratic oath or a face to face encounter and who is distinctly influenced by the quarterly report, meeting targeted economic objectives, and maximization of executives' bonus. Tolerant, detached, relativistic, and non-religious characterizes the postmodern ethos. These traits are hardly unique to the United States but are found in the new global secular culture throughout the world. However, the U.S. is one of the few countries that lacks a national healthcare system and that has influenced greatly the growth of expenditures, healthcare disparities, and other problems.

SUMMARY

In the twenty-first century corporations will have a major role in the conduct of medical practice. However, we should follow Bauman's dictum to question and to challenge the assumptions of common practice. The nature and structure of corporations as well as their regulation, need to be examined and understood especially from an ethical perspective. Those individuals who lost their health insurance after developing serious illnesses over technical errors in their applications represent the type of problem that develops when business ethics become severely attenuated in the postmodern corporate milieu. The moral voice of medical professionalism must not be drowned out entirely by the remote bureaucratic corporate control of healthcare delivery nor by the weakening of social learning of morality. A pragmatic yet principled ethic of corporate medical practice needs to be developed and communicated by the collaboration of business ethicists, bioethicists, corporate leaders, as well as physician organizations, patient organizations, and of course government leaders. This cannot be done by the private and academic sectors without some government input, but the first step is to recognize the urgency of such an undertaking. Developing consensus on this will be very challenging but ultimately necessary if healthcare is to become a rational resource to the people of the nation and the world. There needs to be a healthy dialogue about the intersectons between the values of medical practice and the business ethics of corporate medicine. Questioning the current, commonly accepted aspects of medical care and medical corporations may be, to paraphrase Bauman, the most important task or at least the beginning of a very important task.

NOTES

1. Robinson J. C. *The Corporate Practice of Medicine*. Berkeley: Univ California 1999, p. 235.
2. Bauman Z. *Globalization: The Consequences*. Cambridge: Polity Press, 1998. Globalization: The Human Consequences

3. Robinson J. C. *The Corporate Practice of Medicine*. Berkeley: Univ Calif Press, 1999, 235.

4. http://www.healthcare.gov/news/factsheets/2011/03/accountablecare03312011a.html. Accessed March 31, 2013.

5. Ibid., 213.

6. Ibid., 214.

7. Sach JD. *The Price of Civilization: Reawakening American Virtue and Prosperity*. Chapter 3. The Free-market Fallacy. New York: Random House, 2011.

8. http://www.gpo.gov/fdsys/pkg/BILLS-111hr3590enr/pdf/BILLS-111hr3590enr.pdf. Accessed November 24, 2012.

9. Bell D. *The Cultural Contradictions of Capitalism*. New York: Basic Books, 1976.

10. Mary H., Michal J. D., Meg S. L., Pekarske J. D., Matthew K. McManus, J. D. Reinhart, Boerner Van Deuren. Corporate Practice of Medicine Survery http://www.nhpco.org/sites/default/files/public/palliativecare/corporate-practice-of-medicine-50-state-summary.pdf. Accessed April 28, 2013.

11. Milliman Inc. http://www.milliman.com/expertise/healthcare/products-tools/milliman-care-guidelines/index.php.

12. http://www.mckesson.com/en_us/McKesson.com/For%2BPayors/Private%2BSector/InterQual%2BDecision%2BSupport/InterQual%2BDecision%2BSupport.html

13. Milliman Inc., Ibid.

14. McKesson Decision Support. http://www.mckesson.com/payers/decision-management/decision-management/.

15. Mitus A. J. The Birth of InterQual: Evidence-Based Decision Support Criteria that Helped Change Healthcare. *Professional Case Management* 13(4): 228–233, 2008.

16. Barlett DL, Steele JB. *Critical Condition: How Health Care in America Became Big Business & Bad Medicine*. New York: Doubleday, 2004.

17. Eddy David. Health Technology Assessment and Evidence-Based Medicine: What are We Talking About? *Value in Health*. 12(2):56–57, 2009.

18. Barlett DL Steele JB op cit., 164–165.

19. Final Matenity Length of Stay Rules Published. http://www.ncsl.org.health/final-maternity-length.

20. Liu S., Heaman M., Kramer M. S., et al. Length of hospital stay, obstetric conditions at childbirth, and maternal admission. *Am J Obstet Gynecol* 187(3): 681–7, 2002.

21. Meredith J. W., Burney R., Burton S., et al. Milliman & Robertson Length of Stay Guidelines Are Not Appropriate for Trauma Patients: A Comparison With the Ntdb. *J. Trauma* 47(1): 208, 1999.

22. Rutledge R. An analysis of 25 Millilman & Robetson Guidelines for Surgery: Data driven versus Consensus Derived Clinical Practice Guidelines. *Annals Surgery* 228(4):579–587, 1998.

23. Bartlett D. L., Steele J. B. *Critical Condition: How Healthcare in America Became Big Bigness and Bad Medicine*. New York: Doubleday, 2004, p. 168.

24. Romley J. A., Jena A. B., Goldman D. P. Hospital Spending and Inpatient Mortality: Evidence from California. *Ann Int Med* 154:160–167, 2011.

25. Sturmberg J. P., Martin C. M. Complexity and health—yesterday traditions, tomorrow's health. *J. Evaluation Clinical Practice*. 15:543–548, 2009.

26. Chuang S., Inder K. An effectiveness analysis of healthcare system using a systems theoretic approach. *BMC Health Services Research* 9: 195, 2009.

27. Lyotard Jean-Francois. *The Post Modern Explained*. Minneapolis: University of Minnesota Press. 1993, p. 122.

28. Issacson Walter. *Steve Jobs*. New York: Simon Schuster, 2011.

29. Eiser A. R., Goold S. D., Suchman A. L. Bioethics and Business Ethics in the Management of Healthcare. *J Gen Int Med* 14: S58–62, 1999.

30. Bethany MacLean, Elkind Peter. *The Smartest Guys in the Room: The Amazing Rise and Scandalous Fall of Enron*. New York: Penguin, 2003.

31. Thomas K., Schmidt M. S. Glaxo agrees to pay $3 billion in fraud settlement. *NY Times*. July 2, 2012. http://wwwnytimes.com/2012/07/03/business/glaxosimthkline-a.

32. Etzioni A., Mitchell D. Corporate Crime. http://www.gwu.edu/~ccps/etzioni/documents/A366.pdf. Accessed February 18, 2011.

33. J. H. Davis, Lerer L. Romney vows repeal of Dodd-Frank. *Businessweek*. May 14, 2012.http://www.businessweek.com/news/2012-05-14/jpmorgans-inconvenient-truth-hits-romneys-dodd-frank-repeal-vowing.

34. Jackal Robert. *Moral Mazes*. New York: Oxford University Press.1988.

35. Ian Buchanan. *Fredric Jameson: Live Theory*. Continum 2006 p. 87.

36. LA Times. Lisa Girion. July 17, 2009. http://articles.latimes.com/print/2009/jun/17/business/fi-rescind17

37. Bauman Zygmunt. Collateral casualties of consumerism. *J. Consumer Culture* 25–56, 2007.

38. D. Yankelovich. Two Truths from the Social Sciences, in Borchert D. M., Stewart D., eds. *Being Human in a Technological Age*. Athens, Ohio: Ohio State Univ Press 1979, p. 103.

39. Eiser A. R., Goold S. D., Suchman A. L. Bioethics and Business Ethics in the Management of Healthcare. *J Gen Int Med* 14: S58–62, 1999.

40. Edward Freeman. *Strategic Management: A Stakeholder Approach*. Cambridge Univ Press 1984.

41. Frederick WC. *Values, Nature, and Culture in the American Corporation*. New York: Oxford Univ, 1995, p. 217.

42. Ibid., 96.

43. Schlesinger M., Quon N., Wynia M., Cummins D., Gray B. Profit-seeking, corporate control, and the trustworthiness of health care organizations: Assessments of health plan performance by their affiliated physicians. *Heatlh Services Research* 40(3): 605–645, 2005.

44. Pulkkinen, T. (1996). *The Postmodern and Political Agency*. Helsinki University, Department of Philosophy. Ph.D. dissertation. Helsinki: Hakapaino.

45. Bauman Zygmunt. *Postmodernist Ethics*. Oxford: Blackwell, 1993.

46. Kelemen M., Peltonen T. Ethics, morality, and the subject: the contribution of Zygmunt Bauman and Michel Foucault to 'postmodern' business ethics. *Scand J Mgmt* 17:151–166, 2001.

47. Ibid., 164.

48. Donaldson T., Dunfee T. W. *Ties that Bind: A Social Contracts Approach to Business Ethics*. Cambridge, MA: Harvard Business School Press, 1999.

49. Cialdini R. B., Petrova P. H., Goldstein N. J. The Hidden Costs of Organization Dishonesty. *MITSloan Management Review*. 45(3):67–73, 2004.

50. Rawwas M. Y. A., Al-Khanth J. A., Vitell S. J. Academic Dishonesty: A Cross-Cultural Comparision of US and Chinese Marketing Students. *J Marketing Education* 26(1):89=100, 2004.

51. Grimes P. W. Dishonesty in Academics and Business: A Cross-cultural Evaluation of Student attitudes. *J Business Ethics*. 49:273–290, 2004.

52. Morris David. *Illness and Culture in the Postmodern Age*. Berkeley: Univ. Calif Press 1998. p. 275.

53. C. Arnst. In Most Markets, a Few Insurers Dominate. Bloomberg Business Week. http://www.businessweek.com/print/magazine/content/09_31/b4141022519011.htm. Accessed February 19, 2011.

54. M. J. McCue. M. H. Bailit. Commonweatlh Fund report.http://www.commonwealthfund.org/~/media/Files/Publications/Issue%20Brief/2011/Jun/1511_McCue_assessing_financial_hlt_Medicaid_managed_care_plans_ib_FINAL.pdf. Accessed Nov 24, 2012.

Chapter Six

Power and Trust in the Patient-Physician Relationship

Postmodern Values and the Patient-Centered Medical Home

"The final word on power is that *resistance comes first*." —Giles Deleuze in *Foucault*[1]

"To discover such an orientation in the I is to identify the I with morality. The I before the Other is infinitely responsible. The Other who provokes the ethical movement consciousness." —Levinas[2]

Postmodern clinical relationships are very different from those in the twentieth century and are marked by increasing complexity in the social structure of medical care. Changes in the social structure of medicine reflect changes in the relative power of patients, physicians and other caregivers as well as the alterations caused by information technology. A highly pertinent example of these shifts is the Patient-Centered Medical Home (PCMH) model of medical care. The PCMH is a newer method of primary care delivery that features a team-based approach that emphasizes coordination of care across the continuum, use of an EHR, collection of quality measures, and, at least potentially, individualizes care according to patient characteristics.[3] In considering early experience with the PCMH model, we should consider whether there are alternatives to clinical care models that may better meet patient needs. I suggest in this chapter that the philosophical observations of Deleuze and Guattari, as well as those of Levinas, offer heuristics that elucidate some of the characteristics of alternative clinical care models to the highly computerized data-focused PCMH. Deleuze and Guattari describe a path to avoid the straitjacket of the case-hardened bureaucracy,[4] while Levinas provides a postmodern philosophy of responsibility for the Other that avoids moral relativism and the impossibility of consensus.[5]

The role of physicians in delivering medical care is increasingly shared with other professional groups, complex healthcare systems, healthcare insurers, and even with the patients themselves. Paternalism is philosophically very *passé*, even though vestiges may remain in some medical practices and in areas where clinical resources and competition are still limited. The relative power of physicians and patients has changed in many ways. Patients now compose their own online ratings of physicians on websites,[6] and these ratings can change the balance of power. Physician and patient may unite in their efforts to get the insurance plan to pay for a new clinical procedure. If the procedure is done and the results are not those desired, the patient may contact her attorney who requests the medical records from the health system and contemplate litigation if personal injury occurred. The health system administrator enters the inquiry into the physician's record of ongoing professional performance review as mandated by the accrediting organization, The Joint Commission.[7] At each step, resistance arises when one or both parties become aware that new actors and actions are changing the power relationship. While Deleuze may be *slightly* exaggerating that the resistance comes first, certainly a constant flux of power changes and resistance is evident in the newly evolving structures of medical care.

The power formerly exercised by physicians is flowing to administrators, national accrediting organizations, patient groups, and other stakeholders in part because physicians are no longer the sole source of authority on medical information and because they are frequently employed by healthcare systems. Proliferation of online blogs and online publications has broken the hegemony of editorial control by traditional medical journals but has also confused healthcare professionals and patients alike with a wide array of contrasting data and interpretations. Control now moves with the instantaneous communication of information. Deleuze calls for "circuit breakers," i.e. vacuoles that elude control.[8] Wikileaks would appear to be another such example of such circuit breaker, computerized but beyond the control of the dominant power bureaucracies. For medical care such circuit breakers include the physicians', patients', and nurses' blogs, online journals and social media.

Consider some of Jurgen Habermas' concepts in order to understand how clinical care has evolved in this postmodern world. Habermas refers to "consensus or communicative oriented actions. "I call *communicative* those actions in which the behavioral goals or plans of actors are coordinated not via egocentric calculations of success but through consensual exchanges."[9] So, in the clinical realm Habermas' concept of communicative oriented actions would replace individual and corporate egocentric calculations—for example, financial incentives—with evidence-based standards of care that are arrived at by a community of investigators and possibly patients as well.

Of course egocentric calculations may influence not only individual clinicians, but also the community of investigators that would form the foundation of communicative oriented clinical care. This community of investigators might have a hidden vested interest that is shared with the sponsors of their research studies. Some clinicians may recall when the recommendation of post-menopausal estrogens was so strong that it took a form of advocacy as it was based on poorly conducted case control studies.[10] Clinicians and investigators were both alternatively chastened and heartened when better analyzed case controlled studies and randomized control trials provided a more complete, complex, and accurate picture of the risks as well as benefits of such treatment.[11] Post-menopausal estrogen usage is but one example of a change in the clinical paradigm that is influenced by tacit power relations until a new equilibrium is achieved. Clinical data is certainly part of the equilibrium but hardly the only influence.

Deleuze notes that not all opinions are equally valid, but the postmodern instinct is to avoid judging one as better than another. However, to practice medicine, judgments must be made and acted upon. Practicing physicians do not have the time to analyze and dissect each new publication for its merits. Physicians must trust the judgment of others to distill all of the latest studies. Patients also need to trust their physicians' recommendations, or if not, to find other sources of medical authority whom they can trust. At some point the patient must agree to something and commit to a diagnostic and treatment plan. Treatment decisions always entail leaps of faith by both the patient and the clinician and even the best guideline is fallible and may be even inappropriate to selected outliers with exceptional qualities.

How can good clinical care be rendered when authority on medical information and treatment options is widely distributed in the complex flux of the social structure of medical care? Solid data, sound judgment, and appropriate experience are all essential to sound clinical decision-making. But at some point there needs to be an agreement or reconciliation among the participants—the patient, the physician, other healthcare professionals, the health systems, and the healthcare insurers. These decisions are often complex and may be beyond a layperson's understanding and sometimes even beyond an experienced professional's understanding.

In order to understand and work with postmodern clinical relationships, it is helpful to consider the metaphor of the rhizome and the tree as conceived by Deleuze, the philosopher and Guattari, the psychoanalyst.[12] The rhizome is a non-hierarchal accumulation of parts that resists organization, stratification, and hierarchy. In biology a rhizome is the branching roots of a plant, a portion of which may sprout into a full plant under the proper conditions. The rhizome metaphorically evokes the "aborification of multiplicities"[13] and implies the notion of self-organizing material systems. This de-centered network is either leaderless or only has *ad hoc* leadership. By contrast the tree trunk represents having a centering "authority" that evokes the image of a hierarchal organization.

It is helpful to extrapolate to the "blogosphere" to see how Deleuze and Guattari's metaphors are actualized. Patient blogs and physician blogs are examples of the non-hierarchal rhizome of networked communication with few rules and limited bureaucracy. Websites have a minimum of central control but also tend to have a minimum of impact as the diffusion of information is also attenuated by the profusion of sites. Contrast the distributed network model of web communication with the hospitalization of a patient, where the rules of multiple centralized bureaucracies intersect. These rules include the hospital bylaws, Joint Commission regulations, state regulations, medical legal policies and procedures, as well as the interaction of a multitude of medical professionals in variety of disciplines. The metaphor of the tree rather than the rhizome may be more apropos to the standard inpatient setting but even this is evolving, and a definitive version has not yet fully emerged.

Medical care has been moving more toward the ambulatory setting, and there practices may be more reflective of the rhizome than the tree. Connections and disconnections exist simultaneously and the structure of ambulatory medical practice is actively evolving. The forms of ambulatory care practice vary greatly. While there are ambulatory standards of care such as those articulated by the National Council on Quality Assessment (NCQA) in their HEDIS standards, they are largely geared to primary care practices.[14] Specialty practices are starting to have defined standards set by centralized bureaucracies as well.

PATIENT–CENTERED MEDICAL HOME: PATIENT CENTERED OR DATA DRIVEN?

The Patient-Centered Medical Home (PCMH) has been conceived as a way to improve the quality of primary ambulatory care, reduce healthcare costs and, incidentally, to improve the status of the primary care physician. That the PCMH has been cast as the "savior" of primary care tells us much about postmodern medical practice and suggests that myth-making is not yet over. A more appropriate name for this particular type of healthcare delivery may be the data-driven clinical care center.

Several PCMH demonstration projects have been undertaken with federal grants, support from the Robert Wood Johnson Foundation, the Commonwealth Funds, and other foundations as well as support from selected insurance companies. Work on the demonstration projects has been very collaborative and it seems that a consensus has emerged, perhaps prematurely, that this is the format that primary care should take in the twenty-first century.

After reviewing the nature of the PCMH and implementing a PCMH practice model, is it possible that the "patient-centered" label may be something of a misnomer? Preliminary studies of this practice type have found that it is less to patients' liking than previous forms of primary care practice.[15] The "patient-centered" label could be thought of as a form of creative marketing, a postmodern trademark. The PCMH is complexly structured to include nurses, medical assistants, midlevel providers, and care coordinators as well as physicians. One catch phrase used to describe the PCMH is that all healthcare providers work at the top of their credentials so that medical assistants may be educating the patient regarding self-care instead of the physician. Medical assistants *may* do a fine job at this, perhaps even better then when physicians formerly did so themselves, but the patient tends to *feel* that they have been "handed down the line," so to speak. Patients also report that the physicians who appear in their physical presence are engrossed in the computer screen and interact less with them *en face*. The face-to-face encounter encouraged by Levinas may be less likely in this form of healthcare delivery than previous forms if only because the computer monitor is now commanding attention.

The PCMH is clearly data-driven and computer-centered. Any discussion of the role of electronic health records and decision support systems in postmodern clinical care must first address our often unexamined assumption that computerization is always beneficial. In public discourse, the benefits of computerization are widely accepted as intuitively obvious. But if the last 30 years of clinical investigation has taught medicine and clinical scientists anything, it is that the intuitively obvious is often *dead* wrong. Thus while the truths of clinical medicine may be relativistic, they are still more firmly grounded in empirical evidence than most of human endeavors. While computerization of ambulatory medicine offers the potential for better care, the potential must be demonstrated, and that has not yet been done conclusively. A recent study of ambulatory healthcare indicated that using electronic health records, even in combination with decision support systems, does not demonstratively improve clinical care and clinical outcomes.[16] In a Canadian study that was one of the first randomized clinical trials regarding a computerized ambulatory intervention designed to improve identification and treatment of risk factors for vascular disease[17] (coronary, cerebral, and peripheral vascular disorders) the investigators found an improvement in some process measures but not in clinical outcomes.

Even without strong supporting evidence, public policy is already being crafted with the assumption that clinical care improvements result from these investments, and that all primary care practices should be pursuing this precise format of delivery.

It is instructive in understanding the postmodern cultural influences on medical care to consider the various stakeholders in the development of the PCMH. Primary care physician groups, notably the American Academy of Family Practitioners (AAFP), the American College of Physicians, and the American Academy of Pediatrics all have initiatives regarding the PCMH. The AAFP has spun off a for-profit company to help clinical practices transform into the PCMH model. This spin-off, called TransforMED, provides consultation and coaching to help PCP practices transform into the PCMH.[18] However, transforming to a PCMH can be slow going, accompanied by "change fatigue," and is often a multi-year process.[19] The National Committee on Quality Assessment (NCQA) has developed scoring criteria to grade the level of PCMH adoption[20] and will evaluate a practice for a fee to see if it meets their standards. The NCQA has broad sponsorship from health plans, pharmaceutical companies, and foundations such as the American Diabetes Foundation and has received input from the aforementioned physician associations. Key features of the assessment include:[21]

a. Patient access and communication
b. Patient tracking and disease registry functions almost assuredly electronic
c. Care management and coordination accessing both clinical and insurance databases
d. Support for patient self-management including electronic features such as secure e-mail communication
e. Electronic prescribing of medications
f. Electronic test tracking
g. Referral tracking preferably electronic
h. Performance reporting and improvement preferably electronic
i. Advanced electronic communications between the patient and the PCMH

Thus, a highly functional *electronic* health record system is a key element to the implementation of the PCMH. Implementation of an electronic health record system becomes a major undertaking all of its own. For example, electronic health record products do not all have the "registry" functions that a PCMH needs to be successful. A patient registry tracks patients by diagnosis and compiles their clinical data into a quality report. Moreover technology and interconnectivity gaps frequently exist among different medical practices where some of the critical information may dwell in another practice's EHR especially when the practices and groups are not already part of a staff model healthcare organization. Such gaps must be overcome to integrate different practices and groups into a PCMH. Such obstacles have also been identified in other nations such as Canada and Australia in implementing an EHR.[22]

Reports on early demonstration projects note that PCMH implementation also requires a great deal of change in the work processes as well as the change in the roles and identity of the care providers.[23] Physicians need to exercise facultative leadership skills, skills that do not arise naturally from current forms of medical education and physician selection. Attempting to implement the PCMH causes much fatigue and even burnout in the participants. Nutting et al. are very frank in their assessments of these problems noting that several physicians especially those practicing for many years find the transition quite difficult.[24] Further insights into the challenges for physicians implementing this complex new delivery method can be gleaned from such medical blogs as Kevin MD.[25] R. Watkins on that website notes that there is a great deal of "bureaucratic busywork," documenting the documentation, so to speak.

Neither is the patient experience entirely positive. J. Smith replying to the above posting on the Kevin MD blog notes the PCMH "suffers from the peculiarly American delusion that more technology is the answer to any problem, even a broken personal relationship between doctors and their patients."[26] He mentions that patients do not like the PCMH because it distances their relationship with their physician because now the team is caring for them and they are communicating less directly with the physician. Another blogger notes midlevel providers and other members change practice sites frequently, which confounds the patients with discontinuities in caregiving relationships.

At the center of the PCMH model is the accumulation and transmission of electronic health information along with the bureaucratic assessment and regulation of medical practice. This is not necessarily an inappropriate approach but it is unproven to be superior to other models of care delivery. The presumption that the digital encoding and bureaucratic control of medical information will improve care dominates the development of this model and belies the "patient-centered" label.

Health policy expert Robert Berenson and colleagues[27] note that the cultural, structural, and organizational changes required by the PCMH may not be achievable in all practice models nor is it necessary for the many healthier patients seen in primary care practices. They are concerned by attributing many new responsibilities to primary care practices in the form of the PCMH may be further stressing an already stressed component of the healthcare system. Michael Barr, Senior Vice President for Practice and Improvement for the American College of Physicians, notes that there are several possible variations of the PCMH, and that there are other payment models that could be evaluated.[28]

Taking the blogs and the articles together, PCMH is a concept that has been seized upon by the multiplicity of the postmodern medical stakeholders: national physician organizations, insurance companies, medical foundations, some academics, some business enterprises, national quality organizations, and federal agencies to reduce costs and improve quality. However, it is largely untested and unproven with regard to these two touted outcomes as well as to patient satisfaction.

In one of our internal medicine resident clinics, we have implemented many features of the medical home and have observed the singular benefits of *care coordination with an insurance health plan* upon the cost savings component particularly when focused on patients who have a proven track record of being high utilizers of healthcare services.[29] If the healthcare[30] plan identifies from their administrative database, their high utilizing patients and provides them with additional resources not generally found in a primary care practice such as delivery of their medication to them and arranging rides to ambulatory visits, then hospitalization rates can be reduced by up to thirty percent. But this is a costly effort focused on "frequent fliers," not everyone in the practice. It requires seamless cooperation with an insurance health plan by a practice, a rarity outside of staff model HMOs such as Group Health of Puget Sound.[31] In fact, Group Health of Puget Sound has reported fewer emergency department visits, slightly fewer hospitalizations, cost savings, and improved patient satisfaction and physician acceptance. However, Group Health of Puget Sound reported that PCMH was a difficult implementation that not all physicians can achieve.[32] Some patients are satisfied with fewer face-to-face encounters with their primary physician particularly if it saves them time. Other patients may not be pleased with that arrangement. Moreover the individual dedication and effort of the care coordinator are essential to a successful program, and that person's willingness to *problem-solve* rather than obstruct bureaucratically is essential to the success of this type of coordination.

PATIENT-CENTERED MEDICAL HOME: POTENTIAL FOR RHIZOMATIC DIFFERENCES

What could the philosophical musings of Deleuze and Guattari do to inform the discussion of the PCMH? Deleuze and Guattari can help us understand that physicians, nurses, and other providers as well as patients all feel to varying degrees the "emancipatory desires" not to be restrained in the pursuit of healthcare from their own perspectives. By contrast administrators, regulatory organizations, insurers, and legislators desire to reshape the clinical encounter into a series of highly controlled data exchanges. Deleuze and Guattari raise the possibility of an awareness of the "homogenizing power of the new world order, that if it gains a spatial reciprocity that suspends the tendency or desire for domination and be operative in a rhizomatic system of non-dominating 'becoming' relationships."[33] Can needed improvements in primary care take other forms than the aforementioned format of the PCMH, which appears to follow a formulaic, bureaucratic approach engendered by the NCQA standards? Are there better models for patients requiring less intensity of care? One size may not fit all well, so a dominant accrediting agency may not help realize an innovative, rhizomatic approach to primary care in the twenty-first century.

What would a rhizomatic system of non-dominating relationships appear like? It may be different at an inner city federally qualified health clinic from a suburban HMO in the Puget Sound area. It may have greater cultural sensitivity to its milieu and be less focused on the processing of computerized data. One size does not fit all in healthcare but standardization of clinical processes with national standards inhibits the development of "rhizomatic vacuoles" of human connection and humane healing.

I would submit that the whole alternative, holistic, and integrative medicine movement is a search for such rhizomatic methods of human health in an environment rich with meaning and emotional support. When over two-thirds of the American population tries alternative medical approaches in a given year,[34] this point should not be ignored in developing new methods of primary care delivery. How can the PCMH provide that when it is focused on data information storage, transmission, and analysis? Some patients may prefer a purely mechanistic bureaucratic approach to primary care and so may be pleased with a data-driven patient home. Others may seek one richer in emotional support and connectedness. Between the extremes some variation may be conceived to be offered to patients. Americans prefer to have their care individualized more than standardized. One thing that is constant in pre-modern, modern, and postmodern times is that the patient wants, to some extent, a human connection with her/his healthcare provider and that requires some personal continuity at the provider level, and a face-to-face encounter without the computer screen obstructing the exchange of human caring. How can the PCMH provide that when it is focused on data information storage, transmission, and analysis. Between these two poles, some variations may be conceived and offered to patients.

FACTORS REGARDING TRUST IN THE PATIENT-PHYSICIAN RELATIONSHIP

Fiscella and colleagues studied factors regarding patient trust in primary care settings using unannounced, standardized patient actors.[35] They found that two factors were most predictive of trust: a) when the physician explored the patient's experience of illness and b) longer encounter length. They also found that "finding common ground" and "understanding the whole person" were not predictive of trust. Seetharamu and colleagues did a qualitative metanalysis of determinants of trust among between oncologists and their patients.[36] They identified four factors determinative of trust in this circumstance a) avoiding humiliating experiences during the medical encounter; b) sensitivity to the power imbalance between physician and patient; c) understanding and responsiveness to the suffering from the illness; d) understanding and responsiveness to suffering from the treatment. However other studies suggest oncologists may infrequently meet such ideal standards. Morse et al. observed that oncologists missed the opportunity to be emotionally supportive ninety percent of the time, preferring to stay with a strict biomedical model.[37] Pollak et al. found similar results with an only slightly better twenty-two percent of oncologists responding to an opportunity for empathic communication.[38] I doubt that oncologists are unique in this regard.

So why in postmodern times are physicians stuck in the modern ethos of the biomedical model when they should be modeling on the biopsychosocial-cultural model that includes being emotionally supportive? And once again calls go forth to proclaim that what is needed is to better educate and train physicians to be more empathetic. However, the evidence suggests that those selected for medical school are not so empathetic and that medical school and graduate medical education tend to reduce empathy.[39] Perhaps medical educators are being unrealistic in expecting postmodern physicians to display a great deal of empathy. Nurses are much more likely to be empathetic than physicians. For example, oncology nurses were found to be more likely to share the experience of suffering with the patients receiving chemotherapy.[40] Moreover, such nurses advocate on behalf of their patients' needs. Another study demonstrated that communicating the news of a cancer diagnosis is better received when a nurse is present at the time.[41] So perhaps acknowledging the importance of a greater recognition of the *nurse-physician partnership* in healthcare will go a long way to resolving this concern more effectively than trying to change the physicians' character that formed a long time before the clinical encounter. Power/knowledge, as Foucault observed, are essentially linked and caring may be a small part of the mix unless a third party, the nurse, is brought more fully engaged into the clinical encounter. Teamwork sounds like a promising development in healthcare delivery but it is not that easy to always accomplish. Actual teamwork training requires an intensive and supervised effort. A review of interventions to improve teamwork among healthcare staff revealed that gains in clinical outcomes are modest. Teamwork itself improves with training and the more longitudinal the training, the greater the improvement. [42]

Postmodern medical care is characterized by changing roles of healthcare providers. Midlevel providers have become an integral component of health-

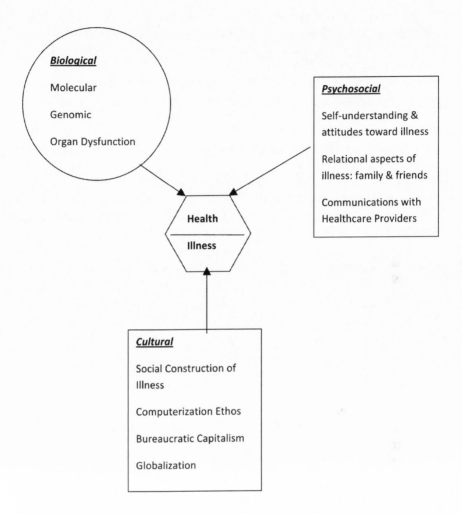

Figure 6.1. Biopsychosociocultural Perspective of Illness and Medical Care

care delivery.[43] However, the roles of other types of healthcare professionals such as pharmacists, physical and occupational therapists, nutritionists, and speech therapists also needs to be considered. These professions have also sought to advance their professional interests by granting doctorate degrees in addition to master degrees.[44] This has created some controversy and confusion as doctors of pharmacy and nursing practice have sought and in some states obtained greater autonomy from physicians in clinical practice. Whether this is advantageous for patients remains to be seen but it will remain part of the postmodern medical milieu.

It is important that physicians in training understand the roles of these other healthcare professionals. Eiser and Connaughton implemented and reported a post-graduate medical educational experience that exposed physicians early in their training to the other "rhizomatic" components of healthcare delivery including visiting nurse services, physical therapy, hospice care, clinical pharmacy, quality improvement, and nutrition.[45] (This educational innovation received the Accreditation Council for Graduate Medical Education (ACGME) Judges Award at the 2006 National Conference). We found residents were more confident and appreciative in working with other healthcare providers when they had seen the work and some of the accomplishments of these non-physician providers. Clearly the practice of medicine in the twenty-first century includes a larger role of non-physicians in allied medical professions, as well as nurse practitioners and physician assistants, but the exact roles and their limits remain to be fully clarified and evaluated.

BUREAUCRACY VERSUS PROFESSIONALISM

One model of the PCMH has it being part of much larger Accountable Care Organizations (ACOs) whose purpose is to reduce healthcare expenditures through reduced hospitalization and greater coordination of care.[46] This involves extensive exchange of data across multiple specialties as well as primary care supported by a digital data network with decision support, standardized order sets, and other means of standardization of medical care. Max Weber's Iron Cage of Bureaucracy is now replaced with a *Silicon Cage* of digital central control and efficiency. The question remains not only whether coordination and cost savings are possible but whether the more humane aspects of clinical care can be preserved or even expanded. As Eisenstadt predicted some time ago, a stable service orientation is based on the existence of a balance between social bureaucratic control and professional autonomy.[47] Giddens posited the notion of more fluid bureaucracies in postmodern institutions characterized by less certainty and rigidity in an era of contingency.[48] Inspired by such optimism about bureaucracies' fluidity, Hoogenboom and Ossewaarde suggest the metaphor of the "pigeon house" of reflexive institutions where controls are characterized by a fluidity of procedures which retain some capacity for subjective perceptions at the professional level.[49] That is not what appears to be developing from healthcare systems and medical education bureaucracies that are determinative today. Is it possible to preserve space for professionalism and human connectedness in the Silicon Cage era, challenging though that might be?

LEVINAS, THE PCMH, AND THE FACE OF THE OTHER

Maintaining a healing relationship among physician, nurse, and patient is seriously challenged by the developing institutions such as the ACO and the PCMH as well as by postmodern attitudes, expectations, values, and processes. The growth of bureaucracy and bureaucratic controls continues with the computerization of medical information, the quality improvement movement and its goal of the standardization of medical care, as well as the improvement of patient safety.

Efforts to maintain the interpersonal aspects of the clinical encounter include the development of narrative medicine, whereby physicians read and write narratives pertaining to their experiences in clinical medicine. The works of Richard Seltzer,[50] Sherwin Nuland,[51] Rafael Campo,[52] and Rita Charon[53] stand out as examples where medical storytelling has reinvigorated the humane aspects of medical practice. However, their influence has been quite limited when compared to the impact of computerization, commercialization, corporate control, and government and quasi-governmental regulation within the healthcare industry. There is a serious imbalance between the narrative and the computerized data.

Emanuel Levinas, building on the earlier work of Martin Buber's *I-Thou*,[54] developed a postmodern philosophy that emphasizes the primacy of the responsibility to the Other. Levinas as a phenomenologist starts with the fundamental nature of human existence—that of dialogical sociality.[55] Starting with the human need for dialogue with other people speaking an intelligible language, he adds the ethical element of responsibility for the Other and notes its primacy, "I am obliged without this obligation having begun in me as though an order was slipped into my consciousness . . ."[56] The focus of the encounter of responsibility is the face-to-face encounter with the Other. It is not the mere gaze but the language exchange that creates ethical awareness of and connection with the Other. According to Derrida,[57] Levinas emphasizes the role of hospitality, an opening of exteriority. He also notes that Levinas's notion of this encounter with the Other also has implications of an infinite transcendence detected through the perceived relationship with the Other. Levinas's conception of transcendence in the relationships with the Other certainly has theological roots. But the emphasis in this context is how this philosophy can relate to the clinical encounter and enrich it. The key here, as Owens notes,[58] is that the power consciousness of clinician and patient be acknowledged to be roughly equivalent, without one consciousness dominating the other. The phrase "patient-centered" is an attempt to establish a power re-equilibration away from paternalism. I prefer a *"dialogic-centered medical home"* where both patient and clinician are aware of the needs for sharing of power and accountability. A far-fetched notion one may argue, however I have had the good fortune to experience it with several patients in my career where patient and physician are there for each other. So I have some understanding that if properly nurtured, it can be realized. As Edith Wyschogrod observes, "Affectivity in Levinas's thought becomes the lived mode of morality."[59] We can care for patients in dialogue rather than glued to a protocol, inputting into an EHR, and concerned about our online ratings.

Perhaps we need to add a reading and understanding of Levinas' insight of the primacy of awareness of responsibility for the Other to an electronic health record, a care coordinator, and portals of medical care to have a medical home where patients and clinicians can feel enthusiastic about receiving and providing medical care. Becker and Robin noted that practice climate correlated well with patient trust in providers where that climate is measured by such factors as delegation, collaboration, patient focus, coordination, and team autonomy.[60] These authors also noted that power in the clinical relationship has favored the physician and that trust is fostered more when the power imbalance is less evident to the patient. We still have a way to go on this path on both sides.

So I ask if the Dialogic Centered Medical Home can engender Levinas' notion of hospitality and responsibility for the Other while keeping with the best aspects of the Silicon Cage in postmodern medical practice? Can a non-dominating bureaucracy in keeping with the Deleuze-Guattari notion of rhizomatic management structures survive in a postmodern corporate milieu? I am suggesting that as the PCMH develops, we need to be vigilant that it does not become a bureaucratic cage of regulation and data storage, retrieval and analysis. Medical leadership will need to ensure that a measure of understanding of the human needs of patients as well those of healthcare providers are taken into account. Primary care may flourish again but it will not do so with a singular focus on computerization, volume productivity, and faceless efficiency. Scales of practice, climate, and patient trust need to be measured as well as productivity and effectiveness. This will require some shift from the present trends that focus almost exclusively on the business aspects of practice that have produced PCMHs where the patients experience the absence of the Other rather than her presence. Physicians will need to assert themselves in the face of greater bureaucratization and corporate control of medical practice that is well underway. Legisiation may be needed to reinvigorate the role of healthcare professionals in the medical practice but that alone will not suffice either. There is a need to raise consciousness of the other dimensions and domains of a dialogic medical practice.

The Dialogic Centered Medical Home will not happen if left only to free-market forces and influences. It will take the raised consciousness of the many providers and stakeholders to foster a new beginning in the twenty-first century to reboot primary care and clinical practice without it feeling to many parties like a Silicon Cage.

SUMMARY

The postmodern development of the Patient-Centered Medical Home (PCMH) is highly computerized, data driven, and largely untested in terms of patient satisfaction, long-term cost effectiveness, and effects on professionalism. Postmodern thinkers Deleuze and Guattari raise the possibility of an awareness of the "homogenizing power of the new world order, that if it gains a spatial reciprocity that suspends the tendency or desire for domination and be operative in a rhizomatic system of non-dominating 'becoming' relationships."[61] Could the PCMH be conceived in a less hierarchal socioeconomic structure? Can Levinas's vision of a dialogic sociality through the face-to-face Encounter of the Other engender a renewed humane approach to primary care? Can the Dialogic Centered Medical Home arise in the postmodern medical practice? These are important questions to consider as we enter the new era of healthcare delivery.

NOTES

1. Deleuze Giles. *Foucault*. Minneapolis: University of Minnesota Press, transl Sean Hand 1988, 89.

2. Levinas E. *Basic Philosophical Writings*, ed. Peperzak A. T., Critchley S., Bernaasconi R. Indiana U Press 1996.

3. http://www.pcmh.ahrq.gov/portal/server.pt/community/pcmh__home/1483. Accessed March 31, 2013.

4. Deleuze and Guattari's BwO in the New World Order. Howard J. S., in DeLeuze and Guattari: New Mappings in Politics, Philosophy, and Culture. Kaufman E., Heller K. J. U Minnesota Press, 1998.

5. Levinas Reader E. Levinas. Edit Sean Hand. Oxford: Blackwell. 1989.

6. Vitals.com http://www.vitals.com/. Accessed November 26, 2012.

7. Ongoing Professional Practice Evaluation (OPPE). The Joint Commission http://www.jointcommission.org/mobile/standards_information/jcfaqdetails.aspx?StandardsFAQId=213& StandardsFAQChapterId=74. Accessed Nov 26, 2012.

8. Kaufman E., Heller K. J. *Deleuze and Guattari: New Mappings in Politics, Philosophy, and Culture*. Univ Minnesota Press, 1998, p. 8.

9. Jurgen Habermas. *The Theory of Communicative Action*. Transl. McCarthy Thomas (Boston: Beacon Press, 1984, 141.

10. Postmenopausal estrogen recommendations reference.

11. Herrington D. The HERS Trial: Paradigm Lost? Heart and Estrogen/Progestin Replacement Study. *Ann Int Med* 131(6): 463–466, 1999.

12. Deleuze G. Guattari Felix. *A Thousand Plateaus* transl. Brian Massumi. Minneapolis: University of Minnesota Press. 1987.

13. Ibid., p. 13.

14. http://www.ncqa.org/Portals/0/HEDISQM/HEDIS%202011/ HEDIS%202011%20Measures.pdf. Accessed January 24, 2011.

15. Crabtree B. F., Nutting P., Miller W. L., Stange K., Stewart E. E., Jaen C. R. Summary of the National Demonstration Project and Recommendations for the Patient-Centered Medical Home. *Annal Fam Med* 8 supp 11:580–588, 2010.

16. Romano M. J., Stafford R. S. Electronic Health Records and Clinical Decision Support Systems: Impact on National Ambulatory Care Quality. *Arch Int Med* 527 Jan 24, 2011. www.archinternmed.com doi:10:1001.

17. Hollbrook A., Pullenayegum, Thabane L., et al. Shared Electronic Vascular Risk Decision Support in Primary Care. *Arch Int Med* 171(19): 1736–44, 2011.

18. http://www.transformed.com/

19. Academy Health. Research Insights. Medical Homes and Accountable Care Organizations. If we build it, will they come? http://www.academyhealth.org/files/publications/RschInsightMedHomes.pdf. Accessed April 30, 2013.

20. http://www.ncqa.org/tabid/631/Default.aspx

21. NCQA. Patient Centered Medical Home Information for practices. http://www.ncqa.org/tabid/1302/Default.aspx.

22. Accenture. http://www.accenture.com/SiteCollectionDocuments/PDF/Accenture_International EMR_Markets_Whitepaper_vfinal.pdf. Accessed November 24, 2012.

23. P. A. Nutting, Miller W. L., Crabtree B. F., Jaen R. C., Stewart E., Stange K. Initial Lessons from the First National Demonstration Project on Practice Transformation to a Patient-Centered Medical Home. *Ann Fam Med* 7(3): 254–260, 2009.

24. Nutting P. A., Miller W. L., Crabtree P. F., et al. Initial Lessons from the Demonstration Project on Practice Transformation to the Patient Centered Medical Home. *Annals of Family Practice* 7(3): 254–260, 2009.

25. S. Wilkins. A Medical Home does not Guarantee Increased Patient Satisfaction http://www.kevinmd.com/blog/2010/07/medical-home-guarantee-increased-patient-satisfaction.html

26. Kevin M. D., Ibid. Comments, J. Smith.

27. Berenson R. A., Hammons T., Gans D. N., et al. A House is not a Home: Keeping Patients at the Center of Practice Redesign. *Health Aff.* 27(5):1219–1230, 2008.

28. Barr M. The Need to Test the Patient-Centered Medical Home. *JAMA* 300(7): 834–835, 2008.

29. Bielaszka-DuVernay C. Improving Coordination of Care for Medicaid Beneficiaries in Pennsylvania. *Health Affairs* 30(3): 426–430, 2011.

30. Bielaszka-DuVernay. Ibid.

31. Reid R. J., Coleman K., Johnson E. A., et al The Group Health Medical Home at Year Two: Cost Savings, Higher Patient Satisfaction, and Less Burnout for Providers Health Affairs. *Health Aff (Millwood).* May, 2010. 29(5):835-43. doi: 10.1377/hlthaff.2010.0158.

32. Meyer H. Group Health's Move the Medical Home: For Doctors, It's Often a Hard Journey. *Health Aff* 29:844–851, 2010.

33. Howard John, S. *Subjectivity and Space in Deleuze and Guattari: New Mappings in Politics, Philosophy, and Culture.* Edit. Eleanor Kaufman, Kevin J Heller. Minneapolis: Univ Minnesota Press. 1999.

34. Kessler R. C., Davis R. B., Foster D. R., Van Rompay M. I., et al. Long-term trends in the use of complementary and alternative medical therapies in the United States. *Annal Int Me* 135:262–268, 2001.

35. Fiscella K., Meldrum S., Franks P., et al. Patient Trust: Is it Related to Patient-Centered Behavior of Primary Care Physicians? *Medical Care* 42(11): 1049–1055, 2004.

36. Seetharamu N., Iqbal U., Weiner J. S. Determinants of Trust in the patient-oncologist relationship. *Palliative and Supportive Care.* 5:405–409, 2007.

37. Morse D. S., Edwardsen E. A., Gordon H. M. Missed Opportunities for Interval Empathy in Lung Cancer. *Arch Intern Med.* 2008; 168(17):1853–1858.

38. Pollak K. I., Arnold R., Alexander S. C. Do patient attributes predict oncologist empathetic responses and patient perceptions of empathy. *Supportive Care in Cancer* 18(11):1403–1411, 2009.

39. Lown B. A., Chou C. L., Clark W. D., et al. Caring attitudes in medical education: Perceptions of deans and curriculum leaders. *J Gen Intern Med.* November, 2007 November. 22(11): 1514–1522.

40. Fall-Dickson J. M., Rose L. Caring for Patients who Experience Chemotherapy–Induced Side Effects: The Meaning for Oncology Nurses. *Oncology Nursing Forum* 26(5): 901–907, 1999.

41. Rossin M., Levy O., Schwartz T., Silner D. Caregivers' Role in Breaking Bad News. *Cancer Nursing* 29(4): 302–308, 2006.

42. McCullough P., Rathbone J., Catchpole K. Interventions to improve teamwork and communications among healthcare staff. *Brit J Surg* 98:469–479, 2011.

43. Jones E. P., Cawley J. F. Physician Assistants and Health System Reform Clinical Capabilities, Practice Activities, and Potential roles. *JAMA* 271(16):1266–1272, 1994.

44. American Physical Therapy Association website. http://www.apta.org/AM/Template. cfm?Section=Post_Professional_Degree&CONTENTID=32362&TEMPLATE=/CM/ ContentDisplay.cfm.

45. Eiser A. R., Connaughton J. Experiential Learning of Systems Based Practice. *Acad Med.* 2008, Oct 1983 (10):916–23.

46. AAFP. Accountable Care Organizations: Can they Rein in Spending for States? http:// www.aafp.org/online/etc/medialib/aafp_org/documents/policy/state/statehealthpolicy/acos.Par. 0001.File.dat/AAFPACObriefJune2010.pdf

47. Eisenstadt S. N. Bureaucracy, bureaucratization, and debureaucratization. *Administrative Science Quarterly* 4/3:302–320, 1959.

48. Giddens A. Living in a Post-traditional society, in *Reflexive Modernization.* U. Beck, A. Giddens, S Lash. Eds. Cambridge: Polity Press, 58, 1994.

49. Hoogenboom Marcel., Ossewaarde Ringo. From Iron Cage to Pigeon House: The Birth of Reflexive Authority. *Organization Studies* 26(4): 601–619, 2005.

50. Seltzer R. *Mortal Lessons: Notes on the Art of Surgery* New York: Simon & Schuster, 1976.

51. Nuland S. *How We Die.* New York: Random House, 1993.

52. Campo, Rafael. *The Poetry of Healing: A Doctor's Education in Empathy, Identity, and Desire.* New York: W. W. Norton, 1997.

53. Charon, Rita, and Martha Montello. *Stories Matter: The Role of Narrative in Medical Ethics.* London: Routledge, 2002.

54. Buber Martin. *I and Thou* New York: Charles Scribner's Sons, 1978.

55. Bergo, Bettina. Emmanuel Levinas, *The Stanford Encyclopedia of Philosophy* (Fall 2011 Edition), Edward N. Zalta (ed.), URL = http://plato.stanford.edu/archives/fall2011/ entries/levinas.

56. Peperzak Adrian, Critchley, Simon, and Bernasconi, Robert. *Emanuel Levinas: Basic Philosophic Writings.* Bloomington: Indiana U Press, 1996, 119.

57. Jacques Derrida. *Adieu to Emmanuel Levinas.* Trans. P. A. Brault, M. Naas. Stanford Univ Press, 1997. Levinas E. *Totality and Infinity.*

58. Owens, Dorothy M. *Hospitality to Strangers: Empathy and the Patient-Physician Relationship.* Atlanta: Scholars Press, 1999, p. 80.

59. Wyschogrod E. *Emmanuel Levinas: The Problem of Ethical Metaphysics.* New York: Fordham University Press, 2000, p. 231.

60. Becker E. R., Robin D. W. Translating Primary Care Practice Climate into Patient Activation. *Medical Care* 46(8):795-805,2008.

61. Howard, John S. *Subjectivity and Space in Deleuze and Guattari: New Mappings in Politics, Philosophy, and Culture.* Edit Eleanor Kaufman, Kevin J. Heller. Minneapolis: Univ Minnesota Press. 1999.

Chapter Seven

Medical Education in Postmodern America

A Physician-in-Training Is a Consumer, Too

"We live in a world where there is more and more information, and less and less meaning." —Jean Baudrillard[1]

"An inquiring, analytical mind; an unquenchable thirst for new knowledge; and a heartfelt compassion for the ailing—these are prominent traits among the committed clinicians who have preserved the passion for medicine." —Lois DeBakey, PhD[2]

"This 'student as consumer' phenomenon and the associated commodification of academic knowledge and thinking have fractured the progressive purpose and function of higher education." —Porfilio and Yu[3]

Honoring the concept of full disclosure, I am not a disinterested observer when it comes to medical education. I serve as the vice president of Medical Education for a medium sized healthcare system and as associate dean of the affiliated medical school. I am also the Designated Institutional Official (DIO), or hospital official responsible for graduate medical education programs, to the Accreditation Council for Graduate Medical Education (ACGME) for the approved residency programs. I was fortunate to receive the ACGME Parker Palmer Courage to Lead Award for DIOs in 2010. Concerned about the present and the future of medical care as well as medical education, I wish to discern the specific postmodern developments that have altered medical education, and how they influence the ethos of medical education and its moral ecology.

The education of a physician has two distinctive components, medical school and graduate medical education (a.k.a. residency training). Medical school only prepares one to enter a residency training program, while residency training usually lasts three to five years, depending on the discipline, and prepares physicians to practice independently as attending physicians. Fellowship training in a subspecialty may follow residency training for one to three more years. Resident physicians generally receive a training license from the state licensure board which indicates that resident physicians must practice under supervision of attending physicians but there is variation by state.

Nearly a third of residents training in American hospitals are citizens of other countries and attended medical school there.[4] A study in the journal *Health Affairs* indicated that foreign born, foreign trained, International Medical Graduates (IMGs) had clinical outcomes as good as American trained physicians and better than American born, foreign-trained physicians.[5] Hence physicians in America are multicultural in both origin and education. Patients in America also come from a variety of ethnic backgrounds, so there often exist differing ethnicities between patient and clinician.

Noteworthy postmodern developments considered in this chapter include 1) how a consumerist ethos has entered medical education and graduate medical education; 2) how simulation may or may not improve medical education; and 3) how these shifts in the medical education process reflect the changing postmodern milieu. Some of these changes may be viewed positively while others raise concerns.

MEDICAL SCHOOL PROCESSES

The vast majority (about 85 percent) of individuals entering medical school matriculate directly out of college, except for those who pursued another career first.[6] Unlike law schools, medical schools do not make a concerted effort for their students to first go out and have work life experiences because of the extraordinary length of medical training, often a decade long. Since medical school alone does not prepare anyone to practice medicine per se, graduate medical education is essential for every practicing physician. Some young physicians have recently noted that one is required to devote a sizeable portion of the "best years" of one's life (20s and 30s) to the serious educational and clinical pursuits of medical graduate and postgraduate education. Moreover, it is a small percentage of the total population of college students who actually seek a career in medicine. Of those who do seek it, 50 percent or less will be accepted into an American medical school.[7] (By comparison, the typical Ivy League college has an acceptance rate of 5 to 15 percent).[8] Those still seeking to become physicians will pursue medicine by attending international medical schools, several of which are located in the Caribbean.

In addition, international medical students from other nations seek residency training in the United States so that nearly a third of physicians entering medical practice in the United States are graduates of medical schools outside the United States. One might inquire why a wealthy nation of over 300 million needs to import physicians from poorer countries. Perhaps a medical career is considered too demanding or not sufficient rewarding for enough American students to pursue it in sufficiently numbers to meet the needs of the American healthcare system. Careers in medicine are usually financially rewarding but the training period is protracted and the responsibilities and stresses are very considerable. Not surprisingly, the crisis in the financial markets resulted in an increase in U.S. medical school applications; applications have risen by almost 20 percent in the past eight years. [9]

What motivates medical students to become physicians? Factors include high income potential, social prestige, job security, opportunity to help others, opportunity to study the human biologic sciences, desire for challenging cognitive and procedural work, desire to work with people in a direct manner, social pressures from parents and spouses, and the opportunity to engage in research. [10] Requirements for admission and completion includes high performance on standardized examinations, grades in scheduled classes, a certain degree of reliability to show up for clerkships and related matters, and the ability to substantially delay gratification for a period of not less than seven years and often more than ten years. The work in careers in medicine and surgery are generally quite demanding and stressful as well as rewarding, challenging, and their products are very significant to other people.

The need to import physicians can be viewed as a postmodern phenomenon evoking global perspectives on economics, social mores, human motivations, geopolitics, and other factors. For one, delaying gratification is *not* a cherished postmodern value. Postmodern uncertainty regarding the future casts delaying gratification as a risky choice. The more hedonistic aspects of postmodern life don't support a decade of delayed gratification especially a decade in a person's life when considerable gratification is possible. The postmodern awareness of potentially cataclysmic personal or world events, such as 9/11, a huge economic depression, a nuclear event, or disastrous global weather tends to inhibit the delaying of personal gratification. A physician's lengthy training constitutes a somewhat risky investment. Often residents today seek more work/life balance during residency than previous generations of physicians did. Moreover authoritative decision-making in healthcare delivery has passed in many instances to non-physicians with the multiplicity of stakeholders in healthcare making numerous demands upon a physician's time and effort. The loss of professional autonomy is also reducing the attractiveness of medicine as a career choice.

The first two decades of a future physician's life is spent quite apart from the world of medicine. Thus when one considers the moral development of a physician-in-training much of that development has already occurred in a social and moral milieu where they are exposed to all the same influences and challenges that future businesspersons, lawyers, and politicians are. In other words, nothing particularly physician-like is present in their early moral development except that individuals self-select for this profession and one would hope that the more ethical and mature candidates pursue a medical career. However, a study by the RAND Corporation found the degree of altruism elicited from medical students was similar to that of business students, although both were greater than that of law students.[11] If the moral aptitude of medical students is no greater than that of business students, then that alone is reason for concern as many parties agree that altruism is a value more central to the mission of medicine than it is to business.

Eiser, Goold, and Suchman noted several years ago that business ethics lack the primacy of medical ethics because the preeminent focus of the business world is return on investment, and the decline in public consensus on socially acceptable norms has significantly impacted the ethos of the business world.[12] So if medical students perform similarly to business students on a scale of altruism then there is reason for concern. Brame, in a forthright reflection on altruism in the last half of the twentieth century, suggests altruism disappears somewhere between the beginning of medical school and the end of residency training.[13] Several aspects of the training itself as well as postmodern cultural changes challenge the development and maintenance of altruism in clinician trainees. In the nineteenth century altruism in medicine in America was closely aligned with the association between Protestant clergy and medical practitioner.[14] It is no accident that the paragon of the modern clinician, Sir William Osler, considered becoming a minister before he chose medicine as his career. Before American medicine had a scientific basis, it had altruism and bedside manner as its principal assets. In the twenty-first century social changes have been wrought not only by advances in science and technology but by a serious rending of the social fabric of American life that was conducive to altruistic tendencies. Grasping for altruism as a foundational concept in medicine may no longer be a realistic possibility. Altruism is rooted in kinship, near-kinship group identity or closely shared living experiences and values, especially religious ones.[15,16] In the postmodern era, heterogeneity, multi-culturalism, pluralism, and social mobility guarantee that the vital ingredients for the flourishing of altruism are going to be in relatively scarce supply. The postmodern ethos favors personal gratification over service to others. Each fall medical educators interview thousands of medical students and observe that the best and the brightest American students pursue the specialties which have the best return on their investment as well as the best work/life balance. These include such specialties as dermatology, radiology, anesthesiology, and disciplines heavy on procedures and short on contact time with patients.

This does not mean that medicine cannot be a moral enterprise. After altruism, there are other ways to invest medicine with moral meaning. Bernard Williams indicated: "Obligation works to secure reliability, a state of affairs in which people can reasonably expect others to behave in some ways and not in others."[17] We can expect reliability from today's physicians if not altruism, but there is unfinished work on creating the circumstances and medical moral milieu that favor *reliability*. Reliability requires a particular type of social milieu as well, and the way postmodern American culture has evolved may not be conducive to reliability either.

Medical school is a competitive environment, not for completing of the course of study, as 97 percent of those starting American medical schools graduate,[18] but to position the graduate for the most competitive post-graduate residencies. Recently I attended a medical conference where the deans of students of several different medical schools concurred that the graduation rate is probably a few percentage points too high. One needs an airtight case for dismissal in the event it is challenged in the tort system. This is the part of the legal system that receives little public attention as the focus persists on medical liability cases after a purported medical error has occurred. But the legal tort system can be used to protect any consumer's interest and that includes the consumers of medical education. A few borderline medical students may graduate despite the faculty's and administration's concerns if the documentation is insufficient to stand up to a court challenge. This conundrum is not unique to any one medical school nor does it disappear during residency training or even during clinical practice after training is completed.

A survey of medical school deans indicates that while their schools encourage fostering a caring attitude toward patients, a number of them note that time and productivity demands on faculty may limit proper role modeling in this regard.[19] So both the outlier and the average student may have a dearth of role models for exemplary professionalism. Another question is whether the group mean has shifted toward the more self-absorbed student, reflecting the postmodern concern for self.

The competitiveness of medical school may engender the possibility of cheating in examinations during medical school. A study thirty years ago (early postmodern era) suggested that over 50 percent of students at two medical schools cheated in some manner during their studies there.[20] A more extensive survey by Baldwin and associates published some 15 years ago, consisting of students at over thirty medical schools, found that 30 percent thought that cheating was a natural outgrowth of medical school competitiveness.[21] Less than five percent admitted to cheating in medical school while over 40 percent of the same students admitted to cheating in high school. Thus it is fair to conclude that there is some cheating on examinations in medical school, it may vary significantly from school to school and student to student, and that it is not a recent development. These studies do raise concern about medical student integrity that may transfer to physician integrity. Only 42 percent of medical students would turn in another student who is cheating.[22] This raises the difficulty of self-policing of medical students. Even an honor code adoption at a medical school may not stop cheating.[23] The situation appears similar with nursing students where between 8 and 39 percent have admitted to cheating at some time while over three-quarters have observed other students cheating.[24] So other respected healthcare professionals also have a desire to seek a competitive edge that raises concerns regarding personal integrity. According to the most recent Gallup poll, nurses are regarded in the United States as the most honest profession while physicians come in fifth, considerably ahead of lawyers and legislators.[25] Despite this checkered history regarding cheating, medical professionals appear among the most respected for their integrity. However, physicians last topped the Gallup list of honored professions as far back as 1976! Thus apparently in the postmodern era, patients (consumers) have discovered the clay feet of the physician "heroes" of the mid-twentieth-century. As I noted in a previous chapter, bioethics and legal developments have recognized the ethical challenges to physicians, both situational and personal. Rodwin, a legal scholar, noted in the era of managed care, financial incentives to reduce expenditures may have compromised the physician's fiduciary responsibility to the patient.[26] He indicated more legal regulation could improve such matters and recommended the establishment of a federal regulatory agency concerning medical practice similar to the Securities and Exchange Commission. I am not sure too many physicians or patients would feel comfortable with such an approach given their low opinion of lawyers and lawmakers noted above. Such an approach also does not address the issue of the physician's moral development nor the social context of honest and reliable conduct.

ACGME AND GRADUATE MEDICAL EDUCATION

The Accreditation Council for Graduate Medical Education (ACGME) is the main accrediting agency for graduate medical education in the United States and thus plays a crucial role in the formation of new practicing physicians in the USA. Simply put if a residency is not certified by the ACGME (or in the case of osteopathic residencies by the American Osteopathic Association), the Centers for Medicare and Medicaid Services (CMS) will not fund the residency training program, while state licensure boards and hospital staffs may not credit the training experience and credential the physician as an attending physician. So these organizations exert *very* substantial control of physician training in the United States.

The ACGME in conjunction with the American Board of Medical Specialties (ABMS) implemented a system of six core competencies: medical knowledge; medical care; medical professionalism; systems based practice; practice based learning; and patient-physician communications. (I had the opportunity and privilege to consult to the American Board of Medical Specialties on the matter of assessing medical professionalism, and to work with ACGME staff on this matter.)[27] Professionalism is the competency most relevant to the current discussion. The ACGME defines professionalism as: compassion; integrity; demonstrating respect for others; placing patients' needs above self interest; respect for patient autonomy and privacy; accountability to patients, society, and the profession; and sensitivity to diversity with regard to gender, age, culture, religion, race, disabilities, and sexual orientation.[28]

With professionalism so broadly and explicitly defined it encompasses cognitive skills as well as personal traits and qualities. The cognitive skills include knowledge about respecting patient autonomy, the fundamental principle of American bioethics, and how to address issues demonstrating respect for the multitude of minority perspectives. The personal traits invoked in this definition comprise compassion, honesty, altruism, and reliability, qualities that are not necessarily part of the medical school selection process nor are they likely to be precisely measured. This wide breadth of the scope of medical professionalism makes it profoundly challenging to foster its development in a group of individuals but especially those reared in a postmodern culture of materialism and personal indulgence.

Huddle takes the ACGME to task for considering professionalism a skill like any other.[29] This author observes that moral norms develop in childhood before higher education occurs. So is it too late to learn professionalism in medical school and residency training? Some of the desirable professionalism traits may begin in childhood but the question is how well are they sustained through the period of young adulthood and the extended period of medical training.

From the social psychology literature, moral development develops primarily in childhood and adolescence and, to a lesser extent, in the early twenties.[30] Huddle points out that the environment in graduate medical education is not an all-encompassing value-laden environment such as a convent or Marine boot camp that is emotionally intense enough to *reshape* moral traits of character. Thus medical schools do not, nor can they, select for moral traits. In addition, they do not exert a great deal of effectiveness at instilling them in the third decade of life.

The ACGME has some operational approaches that may foster the ethos that the resident physician is a consumer of graduate medical education and has a full set of consumer rights. This is the ethical logic of postmodern culture as applied to graduate medical education. The ACGME is being both "politically correct" and concordant with values commonly embraced by educational institutions throughout the United States and elsewhere. It is manifest within the regulations and processes of the ACGME, as it is in other such American institutions under the influence of the consumerist ethos. For instance, the ACGME review committees, in their assessment of residencies, require all of the residents to complete an anonymous survey answering specific questions regarding the program.[31] This unintentionally but inevitably conveys a consumerist ethos to residents in training. The very performativity of a student completing a survey changes the power relationship. Judith Butler indicates that a performative act entails the exercise of speech that has commanding power.[32] Give a resident or student the authority to rate their education and teachers, and this authority will modify the power/knowledge equation. A consumer of education promotes a customer-service relationship[33] that may not be conducive to fostering the accountability needed to be an outstanding clinician.

Reducing the hours that resident physicians work is another major change in GME in the past decade. The ACGME, responding to concerns regarding resident fatigue and patient safety, changed the work hour rules twice, first in 2003 and again in 2011. In 2003, the work hours were reduced to 80 hours a week with one day off per week at a minimum and a maximum workday of 24 hours with partial duties for another six hours. The impact of these rules was mixed. Residents were somewhat less fatigued and their quality of life was improved, while the reduction in fatigue-related errors was balanced out by an increase in errors due to an increase in handoffs, less attendance at conferences, and perceived decreased quality of care.[34] Most worrisome and, in typical postmodern fashion, were the unintended consequences of such a change when studies demonstrated that surgical residents were receiving less training in their specialty,[35] and that residents were feeling less ownership or stewardship of their patients.[36] Rosenbaum and Lamas note that the work hour changes were never subjected to a thorough investigative approach and suggest it is not too late to systematically evaluate these changes.[37] Recommendations by the Institute of Medicine and pressures from Congress led the ACGME to reduce first-year residents' to work a maximum of 16 hours in 2011 and to encourage programs to permit "strategic napping."[38] Inglehart notes the American College of Surgeons expressed "grave concerns" about the latter reductions.[39]

These work hour changes hardly seem conducive to creating the social milieu where a strong sense of professionalism and personal accountability would be expected to flourish. As demonstrated above, no important accrediting agency in America, such as the ACGME, is immune to the postmodern stakeholder pressures exerted upon them. Clearly certain stakeholders have a much greater say in what gets implemented than other less powerful stakeholders. A soon to be published report by the Association of Academic

Internal Medicine notes that 47 percent of program directors in internal medicine have considered resigning that position in the past year[40] and, no doubt, a sense of powerlessness influences such thoughts. The stress of responsibility without authority is spreading among program directors who hold little sway regarding rule changes.

CONSUMERIST ETHOS

"The consumer is always right" may be a useful dictum in consumer retail marketing but how well does it extrapolate to graduate medical education? Do members of society, if they were asked, seek a diminished moral shaping of the medical profession? The 90 hour work week had a boot camp mentality and, as such, was able to shape clinicians values and mores in a way no longer possible. Times change as do social values and medical education like medical practice is not immune to them.

This development is consonant with the critique of Fredric Jameson in *Postmodernism or the Cultural Logic of Late Capitalism* that ethical considerations have been largely replaced by aesthetic ones.[41] He suggests that postmodern culture has mutated under the influence of late consumerist capitalism to derail moral development. Has the ether of consumer rights anesthetized the moral ethos of medical education? If it has, it is part of the general cultural indifference to moral development and not an isolated occurrence. Aristotle described moral development as *phronesis,* an important type of social learning that required making right conduct a habit through practice.[42] The "hidden curriculum" in medical schools and residencies is already a concern for imbuing the incorrect values,[43] wherein attending physicians and senior residents display attitudes of self-interest and sarcasm toward patients and others. My concern here is that consumerist values endorsed by the accrediting agency's policies have inadvertently reinforced another "hidden curriculum," that which inhibits developing a strong sense of personal accountability.

In *The Good Society*, Bellah et al.,[44] note that "the social sciences reinforced the language of utilitarian individualism, and its assumption that social problems are primarily technical rather than moral." While the ACGME core competency of medical professionalism reflects the recognition of the need for physicians to develop a range of moral perspectives, traits, and related cognitive skills, it may be increasingly difficult to fully actualize them. The ACGME is comprised of well-intentioned, highly skilled professionals who are under substantial political pressure to make changes in their policies, sometimes with great haste. For strictly pragmatic reasons, they are also likely to conceive of professionalism in terms of technical skill acquisition rather than as a matter of adult moral development. In the postmodern

ethos, the moral development of its members adapts to a minimalist milieu
for its maturation.

As noted in previous chapters, the prevailing "aesthetic" ethos in medical
practice is focusing now on massive bureaucratic data orientation. Consonant
with this trend, the ACGME is in the process of seeking more electronic
information downloads from each of the 8,000 residency programs under its
new Next Accreditation System (NAS).[45] This will require each residency to
download detailed assessments of each resident to the ACGME website every 6 months so that the organization can confirm it is regularly monitoring
each resident as well as each program.

According to Baudrillard, "Informatizaton is the . . . paradigm of postmodernity."[46] He is concerned about the excessive reliance on the accumulation of data without wisdom. It is no surprise that postmodern medical educational institutions and bureaucracies are not immune to the ideology of "in-
formatization" over older values of hard work, devotion to the profession,
role-modeling, and personal accountability.

Hence the lightness of moral authority in the postmodern lifeworld leaves
an ethical vacuum that bureaucrats seek to fill with data downloads, surveys,
and other forms of information. But can it effectively replace the virtues and
phronesis once learned from parents, religious leaders, teachers, medical
school professors and other cultural and moral role models? There is considerable doubt that the technical bureaucracy can meet the normative needs that
professionalism and personal and public virtues once did. Kultgen, speaking
of professional schools in general, noted that individuals voluntarily join a
profession already possessing a well-formed character.[47] Professional
schools and professional associations may promulgate professional values
but these influences are limited by the "informal curriculum" as well as the
pre-formed character of its members. Moreover studies indicate that for the
most part moral development during medical school is modest at best and
regressive at worst.[48,49] In fact in a more recent study self-interest appeared
to increase, so on a Kohlbergian scale of moral reasoning[50] one could find a
decline in this Neo-Kantian value scale. This may be as the authors of that
study indicated a "hidden curriculum" of self-interest or merely the reality
that postmodern life in all its manifestations in consumerist culture tends to
dampen the Neo-Kantian ideals of universalizable values. Postmodernism
implies a weakening of Kantian and Kohlbergian universalistic values.

SIMULATION IN MEDICAL EDUCATION

Based on the interest in and value accorded to information technology, it
should be no surprise that computerized simulation of medical illness and
treatment is now an important and growing trend in medical education. The

potency of computer technology has permitted the development and marketing of advanced simulation laboratories for a variety of educational purposes
including anesthesiology,[51] resuscitation,[52] and obstetrics.[53] The full extent
of its potential is still uncertain as most studies done so far are short term. It
seems to offer a great deal to medical education with the ability to simulate
clinical conditions without a real patient involved. Once again there is an *a
priori* assumption that it will improve medical education strictly because it is
a technological advancement. Some authors have suggested caution in embracing this modality of education. Wenk et al. note that simulation-based
education is not superior to problem-based learning and raises the additional
concern that participants that used simulation overestimated the extent of
their clinical skill acquisition.[54] The effects of simulated learning are only
beginning to be studied so it may prove to be very valuable, especially in the
more regimented disciplines such as anesthesiology. However, Sierles cautions that the move toward simulation and away from direct supervision with
actual patients may be part of the commercialization and commodification of
medical education in parallel with the commercialization of clinical care.[55]
The Wenk study raises concerns regarding unintended consequences of simulation creating a false sense of competency. This is not to say that simulation will not aid medical education only that it has the potential to create new
concerns. Moreover, it creates new challenges to the narrative aspects of the
clinical encounter that are so important both in the moral development of the
physician as well as to the actual caring for patients.

In *Simulacra and Simulation*, Baudrillard raises another concern with
regard to simulation and illness. He raises the issue that the patient can
simulate some symptoms, and the physician is not prepared to practice medicine with the uncertainty of simulated symptoms mixing with "real" symptoms.[56] Thus simulation may be used by the patient as well as the medical
educator. The potential for simulation to confuse the physician trainee is
compounded by the multi-media nature of medical education today. Consider
Erikson's insight: "Put differently: when growing amounts of information are
distributed at growing speed, it becomes increasingly difficult to create narratives, orders, and development sequences. The fragments threaten to become hegemonic. This has consequences for the ways we relate to knowledge, work, and lifestyle in a wide sense."[57] So too the use of simulation
instead of direct patient interaction may cause a fragmentation of medical
knowledge and a disjunction in communication that may inhibit developing
the full narrative that patient care has always meant in the clinical encounter.
Bauman, in *The Hurried Life or Liquid Modern Challenges to Education*,
emphasizes that consumerist society is hurried, focused on instant gratification, manufactures uncertainty to create dependence on information connectedness, and blurs cultural values that develop over a period of time.[58] The
values of medical professionalism require durability of relationship, individ-

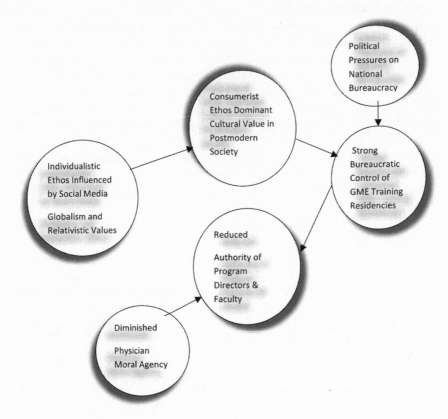

Figure 7.1.   Medical Education and the Consumerist Ethos

ual accountability, integrity, and constancy of meaning. All these qualities are seriously challenged by the features of postmodern culture that are evident to those willing to discern these developments in our society. These are further intensified by the very strong push by both government and private organizations to electronically digitize medical record and information. Digital data has an effect on human beings apart from its content and may further push clinical practice and medical education away from the humanistic approaches as the narrative gets lost in the data downloads.

A POSSIBLE CAUSE OF UNPROFESSIONAL CONDUCT: ELECTRONIC SENSORY OVERLOAD

Consider the report from seventy-eight American medical schools that the incidence of online unprofessional behavior by medical students is common and includes violations of patient confidentiality, profanity, discriminatory language, depiction of intoxication, and sexually suggestive material.[59] The authors conclude that many medical schools lack an adequate policy to deal with electronic misconduct at all. Fewer than 10 percent of the seventy-eight medical schools participating suspended or dismissed the students guilty of such infractions. However many have now caught up with the need for an online professionalism set of policies to prevent such inappropriate content in the electronic media.

Why is there such an underwhelming response by the administrations? It is fair to suggest that this is indicative of the thinness of moral values in the consumerist ethos of postmodern American higher education. The medical student is a consumer with consumer rights and pays high tuition fees. Why is this happening now? This generation of medical students is the first to grow up with computers, smart phones, and other electronic accoutrements. Willard noted that cyberspace creates a communication milieu where hurtful communication is committed without the sender receiving strong affective feedback. She asks appropriately, "Does humankind have the capacity as a species, to expand our moral reasoning, moral motivation and moral control capabilities to deal with the complexities of the information age?"[60] Neuroscientists have also made similar observations. Greenfield at Oxford University is concerned about the way electronic sensory experiences are changing the way personal identity is constructed and notes that this leads to a degree of depersonalization.[61] Immordino-Yang and Damasio, of the Brain and Creativity Institute at the University of Southern California, note that the hyper-speed of computer technology information does not permit adequate time for moral judgment to develop.[62] Dossey notes that the subtle, almost invisible influences of the profusion of electronic media may have a negative influence on the current generation and that we need to be more mindful of it.[63] I believe this phenomenon explains much of the amoral/immoral conduct online by the medical students as described above. No one intended this effect of information technology; it is another unintended consequence. But that does not mean it doesn't have an important effect on postmodern culture. Jain and Cassel ask whether the U.S. public views the physician as virtuous (knights), self-interested (knaves), or pawns (controlled by institutions and corporations), and cautions both the public and physicians to examine their own accountability and accuracy in the assessment.[64] I would add my observation that physicians are all of the above (knights, knaves, and pawns), and a consumerist ethos and electronic desensitization account for much of the less desirable conduct.

SUMMARY

Medical education occurs with young adults in a competitive environment. Several of them have admitted to having cheated at some time during their academic career which bespeaks of a societal weakening of moral codes. The ACGME which accredits post-graduate medical education, gives the trainee a considerable role in providing a judgment of their own educational experience through their annual online assessment as well as on-site inspections. The consumerist ethos that engenders such a policy limits the moral authority of the residency directors and faculty. The lightness of postmodern moral authority is evident in this regard.

Medical simulation may help learning in specific regimented tasks but may also add to the "liquid modern" attenuation of longitudinal moral development during medical education. Neuroscience may have a partial explanation for the postmodern lightness of morality that unprofessional online behavior by medical students and resident physicians has glaringly called to the attention of those seriously concerned about the ethical practice of medicine in the twenty-first century. Ethical practice of medicine is still possible but only if we attend to the social and ethical terrain that we now inhabit and seek remedies for its moral thinness. The need to develop thicker moral codes or other solutions (applications) in the postmodern era will be considered subsequently.

NOTES

1. Baudrillard, J. P. *Simulacra and Simulation.* Trans. Glasser, Sheila F. Ann Arbor: University of Michigan Press. 2008.

2. Debakey L. The Doctors Page http://www.doctorspage.net/quotes.asp

3. Porfilio B. J., Yu T. Student as Consumer. *J. Critical Educ Policy Studies* 4(1): March 2006.

4. Salsberg E. S., Forte G. J. Trends in the Physician Workforce, 1980–2000. *Health Affairs* 21(5):165–173, 2002.

5. Norcini J. J., Boulet J. R., Dauphinee W. D., et al. Evaluating the Quality of Care provided by Graduates of International Medical Schools. *Health Affairs* 29(8): 1461–1468, 2010.

6. https://www.aamc.org/download/64326/data/msq2008.pdf.

7. Association of American Medical School website: https://www.aamc.org/students/considering/85114/gettingin/.

8. Tanya Abrams. 7 of 8 Ivy League Schools Report Lower Admission Rates. NY Times. Accessed May 3, 2013.

9. AAMC. https://www.aamc.org/download/153708/data/charts1982to2012.pdf. Accessed December 2012.

10. Vaglum P., Wiers-Jensssen J., Ekeberg O. Motivation for medical school: the relationship to gender and specialty preferences in a nationwide sample. *Medical Education* 33:236–242, 1999.

11. Coulter I. D., Wilkes M., Martirosian C. Altruism revisited: a comparison of medical, law and business students. *Med Education* 41(4): 341–345, 2007.

12. Eiser A. R., Goold S. D., Suchman A. L. The role of bioethics and business ethics. *J Gen Int Med* 14(suppl1): S558–S62, 1999.

13. Brame R. G. What Happened to Altruism? *Ob Gyn* 112: 687–688, 2008.

14. Imber J. B. *Trusting Doctors: The Decline of Moral Authority in American Medicine.* Princeton, NJ: Princeton Univ Press, 2008.

15. Bowles S. Group Competition, Reproductive Leveling, and the Evolution of Human Altruism. *Science* 314:1569–1572, 2006.

16. Wade N. *The Faith Instinct: How Religion Evolved and Why It Endures.* New York, Penguin Press. 2009, 69–70.

17. Williams B. *Ethics and the Limits of Philosophy.* Cambridge, Mass: Harvard Univ Press 1985, p. 187.

18. AMA News. http://www.amednews.com/2012/03/19/prrb0319.htm, accessed May 3, 2013.

19. Lown B. A., Chou C. L., Clark W. D., et al. Caring attitudes in medical education: Perceptions of Deans and Curriculum Leaders. *J Gen Intern Med* 22(11): 1514–1522, 2007.

20. Sierles F. S., Hendricks I., Circle S. Cheating in Medical School. *J Med Educ.* 55:124–125, 1980.

21. Baldwin D. C. Jr., Daugherty S. R., Rowley B. D., Schwarz M. D. Cheating in medical school: a survey of second-year students at 31 schools. *Acad Med* 71(3): 267–273,1996.

22. Ibid.

23. Sierles F. S., Kushner B. D., Krause P. B. A Controlled Experiment with a Medical Student Honor System. *J Med Educ* 63: 705–712, 1988.

24. Brown D. L. Cheating Must be Okay—Everybody Does It! *Nurse Educator.* 27(1): 6–8, 2002.

25. Gallup Poll Dec 3, 2010 http://www.gallup.com/poll/145043/nurses-top-honesty-ethics-list-11-year.aspx?version=print.

26. Rodwin M. A. *Medicine, Money, and Morals.* New York: Oxford Univ Press, 1993, p. 239.

27. Lynch D. C., Surdyk P. M., Eiser A. R. Assessing Professionalism: A Review of the Literature. *Medical Teacher.* 2004, Jun 26(4):366–7.

28. ACGME website: http://www.acgme.org/outcome/comp/GeneralCompetenciesStandards21307.pdf

29. Huddle T. S. Teaching Professionalism: Is Medical Morality a Competency. *Acad Med* 80 (10): 885–891, 2005.

30. Turiel E. *The Development of Social Knowledge: Morality & Convention.* New York: Cambridge University Press, 1993.

31. ACGME Common Requirements. http://www.acgme.org/acgmeweb/Portals/0/PDFs/commonguide/CompleteGuide_v2%20.pdf Accessed May 5, 2013.

32. Butler Judith. *Bodies that Matter: On the discourse of sex.* New York: Routledge, 1993.

33. Delucchi M., Smith W. L. A Postmodern Explanation of Student Consumerism in Higher Education. *Teaching Soc.* 25:322–327,1997.

34. . Desai S. V., Feldman L., Brown L., et al. Effect of the 2011 vs 2003 Duty Hour Regulation-Compliant Models on Sleep Duration, Trainee Education, and Continuity of Patient Care among Internal Medicine House Staff. *JAMA Intern Med* 2013: 1–7.

35. Nakayam D. K., Taylor S. M. SESC Practice committee survey: Surgical practice in the duty-hour restriction era. *Ann Sur* 79(7): 711-5, 2013.

36. Churdgar S. M., Cox C. E., Que L., et al. Current teaching and evaluation methods in critical care medicine: Has the Accreditation Council for Graduate Medical Education affected how we practice and teach in the intensive care unit? *Crit Care Med* 37:49-60, 2009.

37. Rosenbaum L., Lamas D. Resident Work Hours-Toward an Empirical Narrative. *N Engl J Med* 2012; 367:2044–2049.

38. Iglehart J. K. The ACGME's Final Duty-Hours Standards—Special PGY-1 Limits and Strategic Napping. *N Engl J Med* 363:1589–1591, 2010.

39. Ibid.

40. Personal communication.

41. F. Jameson. *Postmodernism or the Logic of Late Capitalism.* Verso: 1991.

42. Aristotle Phronesis in *Nicomachean Ethics* in *The Complete Works of Aristotle*, (Bollingen Series; 71:2) ed. by Jonathan Barnes, Princeton: Princeton University Press, 1984.

43. Hafferty F. W., Franks R. The hidden curriculum, ethics teaching, and the structure of medical education. *Acad Med* 69(11):861–871, 1994.

44. Bellah R. N., Madsen R., Sullivan W. M., et al. *The Good Society* New York: Knopf, 1991, p. 163.

45. Nasca T., Phillbert I., Brigham T., Flynn T. C. Next GME Accreditation System. *N Engl J Med* 2012; 366:1051–1056 .

46. Dean J. "The Networked Empire: Communicative Capitalism and the Hope for Politics" in *Empire's New Clothes* ed. Passavant PA, Dean J. New York: Routledge, 2004, p. 266.

47. Kultgen J. *Ethics and Professionalism.* Philadelphia: Univ of Penna Press, 1988, p. 366.

48. Self D. J., Schrader D. E., Baldwin D. C. The moral development of medical students: a pilot study of the possible influence of medical education. *J Med Educ* 27:26–34, 1993.

49. Patenaude J., Niyonsenga T., Fafard D. Changes in students' moral development during medical school: A cohort study. *Can Med Assoc J* 168(7):840–844, 2003.

50. Kohlberg L. (1973). The Claim to Moral Adequacy of a Highest Stage of Moral Judgment. *Journal of Philosophy* (18): 630–646. http://en.wikipedia.org/wiki/Digital_object_identifier

51. Cumin D., Merry A. F. Simulator use in anaesthesia. *Anaesthesia.* 62(2):151–162, 2007.

52. Cooper J. B., Taqueti V. R. A brief history of the development of mannequin simulators. *Qual Safety in Health Care* 13(1): i11–i18, 2004.

53. Jude D. C., Gilbert G. G., Magrane D. Simulation training in obstetrics and gynecology clerkship. *Amer J Obstetrics Gyn* 195 (5): 1289–1492, 2006.

54. Wenk M., Waurick R., Schotes D., et al. Simulation-based medical education is no better than problem-based discussions and induces misjudgment in self-assessment. *Adv Health Sci Educ* 14:159-171, 2009.

55. Sierles F. The Revolution is Upon Us. *Acad Med* 85(5): 799–805, 2010.

56. Baudrillard J. *Simulacra and Simulation.* Transl. Glaser SF. Ann Arbor: U Mich Press, 1994, p. 3.

57. Eriksen T. H. *Tyranny of the Moment: Fast and Slow Time in the Information Age* London: Pluto Press, 2001, p. 109.

58. Bauman Zygmunt. *Does Ethics Have a Chance in a World of Consumers* Cambridge, MA: Harvard U Press, 2008. Chapter 4, Hurried Life or . . . or Liquid Modern Challenges to Education. Pp. 144–193.

59. Chretien K. C., Greysen S. R., Chretien J.-P., Kind T. Online Posting of Unprofessional Content by Medical Students. *JAMA* 302(12): 1309–1315, 2009.

60. Willard N. Moral Developments in the Information Age. http://tigger.uic.edu/Moral Ed/articles/willard.html

61. Greenfield S. Reinventing human identity. *New Scientist.* 2656:48.49, 2008.

62. Immordino-Yang M. H., McColl A., Damasio H., Damasio A. Neural correlates of admiration and compassion. *Proc Natl, Acad Sci USA*, 106: 8021–8026, 2009.

63. Dossey L. Plugged In: At What Price? The Perils and Promises of Electronic Communication. *Explore.* 5(5):257–261, 2009.

64. Jain S. H., Cassel C. K. Societal Perceptions of Physicians: Knights, Knaves, or Pawns? *JAMA* 304(9):1009–1010, 2010.

Chapter Eight

Medical Professionalism

What Does Altruism Have to Do with It?

"The practice of medicine is an art, not a trade; a calling, not a business; a calling in which your heart will be exercised equally with your head." —Sir William Osler [1]

"Every man must decide whether he will walk in the light of creative altruism or in the darkness of destructive selfishness." —Martin Luther King, Jr. [2]

DIFFERENCES IN PROFESSIONALISM IN THE TWENTIETH CENTURY

Before considering what the status of medical professionalism is in the twenty-first century, it is important to understand aspects of professionalism in the twentieth century. When Talcott Parsons wrote about the physician's role at the middle of that century, he noted that physicians were viewed as especially valued members of the community, but they were not particularly wealthy. [3] In the 1950s automobile mechanics would actually charge physicians *less* than others, attesting to the fact that that physicians brought value added to the community beyond the financial remuneration they earned. There was a communitarian view of the physician's role in a more homogenous society than in today's consumerist, multicultural environment. Many physicians then considered their uncommon profession a calling which demanded considerable self-sacrifice as well as sacrifice by their spouses and families. This calling may have had, at times, religious overtones. It certainly did for Sir William Osler, a founder of the modern practice of medicine based on accurate diagnosis and empirical evidence at the beginning of the twentieth century.[4] Osler himself was considering becoming a minister until he decided upon a career in medicine. His religious values likely influenced his moral values and his sense of medical professionalism and he in turn influenced generations of physicians. Physicians of the early twentieth century found their patients, patients' families, nurses, and medical students respectful of their skills and responsibilities and of the sacrifices they made to become and serve as physicians. The social contract for physicians in the early twentieth century called for respect for the profession in return for self-sacrifice in providing clinical care. Even though their skills and instruments did not match what clinical medicine can accomplish in the twenty-first century, the respect they were accorded was considerably greater than now. Significant changes in several aspects of society as well as the nature of medical practice in the last quarter of the twentieth century have no doubt altered that aspect of the clinical encounter. The twenty-first century has seen the cultural effects of postmodernism solidify and suffuse, altering the patient-physician relationship.

Another physician motivation that extended well into the second half of the twentieth century consisted of the pursuit of clinical excellence in a competitive environment wherein many of the rewards and incentives were initially non-pecuniary such as the admiration of colleagues, nurses (some of whom became spouses of physicians), and others in the community whether in academic or clinical spheres. The societal pact with the physician then accorded them prestige, respect, deference in clinical decision-making, professional courtesy among one another, privileged parking spaces, exemption from jury duty, and other privileges granted them then but are no longer extended to them. Postmodern culture has changed most of those circumstances in "leveling the playing field," decelerating the physician's social and power status. By revealing the myths of the physician and constricting the physician's decision-making authority, bioethics has contributed significantly to a less exulted view of physicians. Certainly the print and electronic media have also contributed to the declining status of physicians as the several sensational instances of physicians' misconduct were more likely to become news stories than the more numerous instances of their diligence and accountability. If perception on this matter is reality, there is an even bigger problem than I believe.

POSTMODERN VALUES AND PROFESSIONALISM

Five aspects of postmodern culture are particularly worthy of attention with regard to the nature of medical professionalism: consumerism, egalitarianism, multiculturalism, bureaucratic administration, and computerization. In this chapter, I focus on the first two.

Consumerism: As consumerism and the power of persuasion through advertising have grown, the individual (healthcare) consumer becomes the standard unit of value rather than the community. What one consumes becomes paramount in one's life and self-identity. Healthcare became an advertised commodity, like any other, when regulations and traditions pertaining to medical advertising were loosened. Moral ambivalence grew as well as corporatization spread throughout the healthcare industry, and physician productivity became measured in relative value units by corporate bureaucrats.[5] As noted in previous chapters, the patient-physician relationship has changed as a result of postmodern consumerism, and apparently so have the physician values of self-sacrifice and personal commitment.[6] Respect for others and ultimately for the self are marginalized by monetization. The myth of the unerring physician has been replaced by the myth of the unerring market, but that does not necessarily enhance the patient's perspective. The disenchantment of narratives, a major theme of Lyotard,[7] has diminished the role of the physician in the eyes of the patient as care has become technology driven, and human relations in medicine have been diminished by time pressures specialization, and corporatization. The narrative of the ever-ready, ever-caring humanistic physician, *a la* Marcus Welby[8] is gone with the second half of twentieth century. Corporatization of medical care demands predictability, calculability, and control through bureaucracy and computer technology. As the venerable healthcare economist Eli Ginzberg observed a quarter of a century ago, "certain ineluctable forces have drawn medical care into the vortex of the money economy where management techniques must aim at the preservation and enhancement of capital."[9] In some now distant past, the skills of the physician were rewarded with both non-monetary and financial means. But now in the "vortex of the money economy," the non-monetary rewards have further diminished as physician incomes rose. Thirty or forty years ago patients brought their physicians modest gifts and mementos to show their appreciation. Now a physician is appreciative if the patient gives him/her a good online evaluation and does not sue or complain to a medical bureaucracy about the services rendered. When the patient-physician encounter becomes increasingly a mercantile exchange, gratitude drops out of the relationship.

Corporatization and bureaucratization go hand-in-hand with administration via a computerized database. The patient-physician relationship has given way to care managed from afar by a corporate bureaucracy through practice guidelines, order sets, and clinical pathways. This development may have certain benefits regarding measured processes but human relationships are likely to be adversely impacted by bureaucratization of care. Pharmaceutical companies as well as medical product manufacturers seek to have their own influence in the clinical realm so as to maximize their profits. Marcia Angell, former editor-in-chief of the highly regarded *New England Journal of Medicine*, has elucidated the power of such companies to influence which clinical research gets done, how the studies may be biased by such influence, and how this can impact medical education and medical practice.[10] The process of influence is most effective when it is subtle.

Physicians may think they are independent of this process, but even if they are not directly benefitting financially from industry, all are affected since industry funds the vast majority of clinical research studies, major medical journals through advertising revenue, and continuing medical education activities.[11] The need to survive (and thrive) economically drives much of the clinical research and clinical practice in the direction that the industry prefers. The physician becomes a consumer of the industry largesse or at least their clinical trials results. The former is more explicit while the latter is often quite subtle.

Egalitarianism: In its postmodern version egalitarianism seeks equality of gender, ethnicity, and social class but goes further to seek flattening of social hierarchies including medical ones. This flattening of the medical hierarchy has considerable virtue in such settings as the operating room where someone with lower rank may now be able to stop a process left out of a safety checklist in a manner learned from the aviation industry.[12] However flattening of hierarchy may also have a negative effect when it empowers technicians or medical trainees to take shortcuts without facing the repercussions that were more predictable in the more hierarchal past. Since trainees are now viewed as consumers of medical education with rights as well as responsibilities the balance in this regard is important, and it is challenging to maintain in a very precise fashion in an environment of changing roles. Decline in the respect for the medical hierarchy may diminish the role of the mentoring process that was so important in shaping professional values and virtues in prior generations of physicians. When commenting on the character of the present generation, a leader in medical education, research, and practice commented to me that the Baby Boom generation was the most proactive one both when they were at the bottom of the hierarchy as well as when they rose to the top of it. Physicians from later generations, Generation X and Millennials, may already feel less motivated or empowered to influence the course of healthcare change.

The flattening of hierarchy also alters the patient-physician relationship. Patients may be more likely to secure information on the Internet including from patient blogs[13] and challenge the physician's recommendations more than ever before. While this may have benefits in some instances, it may create discord in the patient-physician relationship. The erosion of trust in physicians is well known and growing.[14] In addition to web-based information, patient advocacy groups communicate on web boards raising both a sense of advocacy but also sharpening critical awareness, a true postmodern virtue. Online critiques may engender a sense of solidarity among patients, but it is not too likely to enhance interpersonal dialogue among patient and physician. Gerber and Eiser described patient types with regard to Internet information and participating decision-making: the informed decision maker: the patient who desires both knowledge and authority and the knowledge acquirer who seeks knowledge but prefers the physician to still exert authority in the medical decision-making process. We also suggested the physician might provide the patient with an "Internet prescription" of reliably informative websites.[15] Now patients also communicate directly with one another on patient blogs and form opinions independent of their clinicians. The opinions expressed in a clinical encounter could get repeated in an exchange on a patient blog. Clearly physician authority is going to continue to be challenged in a postmodern, information-rich, flattened hierarchal environment.

CHANGING PHYSICIAN CHARACTERISTICS AND DECLINING ALTRUISM

Moreover increasingly patients are cared for by a group of physicians who may or may not be highly communicative with one another. Examples from the ICU suggest that different medical specialists are not always synchronized with one another in their approach to patient care.[16] There is a complex nexus of relationships including interactions with the insurance companies that alter patient-physician relationships. Trust in the physician is also a powerful predictor of patient satisfaction[17] and patient satisfaction is an important healthcare measure for insurance companies and other stakeholders.

Disciplinary action against physicians by state licensure boards increased 6 percent in 2009.[18] This may represent an actual increase in misconduct or an increased number of complaints by patients in an era of reduced trust and a weaker social contract between physician and patient. Cruess, Johnston, and Cruess, leading authors on medical professionalism in Canada, indicate that societal attitudes toward professionalism are becoming increasingly critical of physicians for pursuing their self-interest.[19] They indicate that physicians need to display altruism to recapture the patient's trust. One must inquire whether altruism is a viable quality in postmodern culture or an archaic concept from a bygone communitarian era.

Several lines of evidence suggest that altruism is in short supply in postmodern medical culture. A survey of anesthesiology educators in Canada using a Delphi method ranked altruism low in a survey of qualities associated with professionalism.[20] Anesthesiology has become one of the most popular choices among American medical students because of substantial income and work/life balance. A survey of medical students in Minnesota found the majority (60-70 percent) consider the quality of altruism problematic.[21] Some residents in internal medicine report difficulty in being sensitive to patients as well as witnessing lapses in professionalism concerning being respectful of others including patients.[22] Bishop and Ross find the term "altruism" unhelpful in today's milieu because of the inscrutability of motive that altruism implies and prefer the "concept of pro-social behavior."[23] Frankly I do not think changing the terminology will suffice although focusing on more measurable parameters may help. It may be time to admit that altruism is waning in our era. After all altruism requires homogenous small group identity[24] and postmodern culture is anything but homogenous. We live in a fast-paced, fact-abundant, image-rich, hyper-technological environment with a multicultural, multi-ethnic, mobile global population.

Roger Jones, a distinguished British physician and educator, wrote of the decline of altruism in medicine in the United Kingdom almost a decade ago.[25] He noted that there is unprecedented public mistrust of the profession fueled by media hyperbole and selective coverage of clinical misadventures. Response to the article was brisk as physicians felt strongly about the reasons for this decline. In personal communication with Professor Jones in 2010, he indicated the decline in the United Kingdom persists and possibly National Health Service rules including work hour rules could be accelerating it.

The decline of altruism is not unique to healthcare. It has been noted that in the postmodern capitalist ethos, where hedonistic values predominate and the sense of communal reciprocity is thin, that altruism is in short supply.[26] Moreover, Jewie Ci[27] points out that a transcendental ascetic ethic is in decline under the influence of capitalism and consumerism. There is nothing to "immunize" physicians or trainees from the larger cultural influences that prevail in postmodern society. One cannot view medical professionalism in isolation from changing values in the society at large.

On another continent, Lipton found that the social status of Australian physicians had changed with the growth of public and private criticism.[28] Several interviewees were nostalgic for the family practioner of the past who made house calls (some even to remote sites by airplane). Many subjects of this focus group described episodes of betrayal of trust by their physicians including medical errors, greed, and even sexual harassment. Many expressed a desire for the physician to be both empathic and objectively competent. Some found empathy more readily from practitioners of alternative medical practices. Those with lower educational levels were more respectful of physicians in general while the well-off and well-educated were more critical of physicians. However, regardless of background, nearly all patients expressed a need for emotional reassurance in the clinical encounter and not merely a commercial exchange for effective medical services. Thus a strict consumerist model of healthcare overlooks the human need for reassurance and caring that is all too often missing in today's bureaucratic model of healthcare.

Postmodern professional relationships are briefer, often lack longitudinal duration, and can be devoid of the emotional content that may have been present in the early and mid-twentieth century when less of the technology of medicine had been developed. It may sadden some older physicians and patients but the younger physicians are not bemoaning the fact as they naturally embrace the new thinner, social pact in the clinical encounter. As Lyotard has observed: the heroic over-arching narratives are no longer subscribed to in this era.[29] As Brame looks back over fifty years in obstetrics and gynecology, he comments that the passing of altruism may have occurred longer ago than we think.[30]

A stunning example of the change in social values and sensibilities is one where first-year medical students at a leading medical school created and posted on YouTube a parody of human anatomical study.[31] Most revealing is that when the medical school dean requested the objectionable video be removed from this social media, these first-year medical students expressed outrage at the infringement of their free speech rights. Thirty years ago one could not technically post publicly such a communication nor imagine doing it without serious repercussions to one's career. Clearly postmodern egalitarianism emboldens the most junior members of the profession to conduct such a tasteless parody and believe it is their right to do so. Burboles notes that parody is a fundamental "trope" of the postmodern education culture and that the greatest risk of the parodist is cynicism and lack of responsibility.[32] Cynicism is clearly a risk to medical professionalism and clinical trust. One can find much cynicism and satire in the entertainment media culture and this attitude filters into the postmodern consciousness where it passes for sophistication.

RECONSTITUTING MEDICAL PROFESSIONALISM

The world has "turned a webpage" into the twenty-first century and there is a need to find new methods to reconstitute medical professionalism. Radical individualism, consumerism, and the power of electronic social media are now dominant while altruism is receding in the rearview mirror but a pragmatic medical professionalism can be reconstructed for the postmodern ethos. Reaching beyond the moral relativism of postmodern multiplicity of values, one can find a subset of values in medical practice derived from clinical encounter outcomes and some basic virtues. Social consensus may thin in general throughout postmodern society, but within the narrow domain of medical professionalism, reconstruction remains possible.

Focusing on the pragmatic and the tactical aspects of patient-physician communications, there are two approaches that may significant improve the clinical encounter: emotional intelligence and mindful medical practice.

Moreover they both suggest methods that can be implemented in medical education.

EMOTIONAL INTELLIGENCE AND EMPATHY

Emotional Intelligence (EI) is both a concept and a set of measurable parameters of behavioral tendencies.[33] This concept, popularized by Daniel Goleman[34] and others, has been studied and accepted more thoroughly in the business realm than in the medical world. Emotional intelligence encompasses self-awareness, self-control, awareness of others' emotional states (empathy), and ability to positively influence others' emotional states. EI varies independently of cognitive intelligence and is a predictor of business success especially regarding leadership.[35] In some instances at least it appears to vary inversely with cognitive intelligence.

The role of emotional intelligence in healthcare delivery is still to be elaborated, as it is very much a work in progress. However several observations have already emerged. A survey of one group of American medical students found that a measurement of emotional intelligence correlated positively with communication skills while it correlated negatively with physical examination skills, which is more a structured cognitive skill.[36] Cognitive measures such as grade point average and standardized aptitude examinations do not correlate with emotional intelligence but EI does correlate with interview scores.[37] Wagner et al. found that patients' satisfaction did not correlate with overall scores of emotional intelligence but did correlate significantly with one subscale on the bar on the EI assessment scale, happiness of the physician.[38]

Perhaps not all components of EI are relevant to the clinical encounter. Empathy as well as physician happiness may be the most important components of EI in attempting to recapture the spark and vitality of medical professionalism. However a study of medical students using the Jefferson Scale of Physician Empathy found empathy decreased during medical school, was lower in male students, and was lower in students who preferred technology-oriented professions.[39]

On the other hand, physician empathy has been slow to correlate with patient satisfaction and compliance, although the correlation is modest.[40] Empathy was also observed to decrease during residency training in internal medicine, and that measurement of empathy is difficult.[41] Yet we know that patients are seeking emotional support from their physicians and often seek alternative or complementary practitioners in order to obtain it. This desire for more emotionally fulfilling and empowering healthcare is evident, and helps fuel the multi-billion dollar alternative medicine industry. Although usually lacking much evidence, alternative medicine has struck a strong emotional response in postmodern Americans.

Technology-driven protocols and practice guidelines can leave patients feeling objectified even when the clinical results are positive, but especially when they are not. Evidence-based medicine requires a focus on the latest studies based on technical information derived from laboratory and imaging assessments and practice guidelines bases on objective information and is analytic in its essence, not humanistic and empathic. So will professionalism in the twenty-first century focus on curing or caring, medical science or medical stewardship? Does it need to be either/or, why not both? If the bureaucracies prevail, humanism and empathy may remain a distant hope. This need not be the case but effort, resources, and leadership will be needed to preserve the humanistic aspects of medical care.

MINDFUL MEDICAL PRACTICE

Mindfulness in medical practice is another approach that engenders compassionate engagement with the patient.[42] Mindfulness is derived from the Buddhist practice of meditation but does not require any particular religious belief. That aspect may be important because young adults today are less likely to express identity with a specific religion.[43] Mindfulness meditation practice heightens awareness of the present moment, permits a disengagement from recollections, beliefs, and emotions, and creates centeredness and equanimity. To the extent it permits one to be fully conscious and aware in the present moment, it can have a liberating effect on the practitioner and can enhance empathic communication with the Other. It can also be important for maintaining the well being of the healthcare provider, physician or otherwise, in a stressful environment. As already noted, a happy, well-balanced health provider is more likely to have a satisfied patient. Anyone who has experienced a disgruntled caregiver is likely to recognize this. Physicians need to heal themselves so they can more effectively heal others. As we have already observed traits like emotional intelligence and empathy appear to decay somewhat during medical training unless a particular effort to reverse this trend is applied. Allen, Wainwright et al. observed that medical training appears somewhat dehumanizing[44] partially due to the nature of medical practice, partly out of the culture of medicine, and partly out of qualities of human nature. Hutchinson and Dobkin[45] at McGill as well as Jon Kabat Zinn[46] caution that mindfulness requires regular practice and that this distinguishes it from other attempts to humanize medical practice although it may be more effective than other techniques. Maintaining a meditative practice is not easy, so this too may have its limits in "humanizing" clinicians; even so, it is certainly warranted to evaluate it fully and carefully as it holds much promise for provider and patient alike. Lutz et al. observed that compassion meditation increased generosity in sharing rewards in a simulation more than cognitive reappraisal training.[47]

What shall motivate physicians to engage in these new methods of humanizing medical practice? Enlightened self-interest is a still a powerful motivation. For example, self-interest can encourage the medical practitioner to demonstrate empathic qualities toward patients because communicating with patients in a respectful, caring manner and tone of voice reduces the risk of malpractice litigation.[48] Moreover, patient complaints against physicians correlate with rates of medical liability litigation.[49] So physicians can avoid both patient complaints about them and the dreaded lawsuit by communicating in an empathetic and caring manner. With advancing medical technology and clinical effectiveness, too often physicians have lost our humility and concern toward patients. Now, out of necessity for a safer medical practice, physicians need to renew the humanistic quality of the clinician through a variety of twenty-first century techniques, even those with ancient roots. Biller-Andorno and Lee caution against excessive reliance on self-interest of physicians as a motivator[50] and advocate for a "shared purpose" motivation. But the thinner moral ethos of postmodernism raises the questions whose shared purpose and how strong is the sharing.

An important study by investigators led by Krasner and Epstein at the University of Rochester School of Medicine found that an intervention consisting of an intensive ten-month program with training in mindfulness meditation, appreciative inquiry, self-awareness exercises, and didactic material on conflict resolution and burnout avoidance led to significant improvements in physician empathy, mood, emotional well-being, and reduced burnout.[51] The authors noted that this was a self-selected volunteer group of physicians so the results may not be generalizable to a less wiling group of clinicians. Parameters such as patient satisfaction and clinical outcomes were not measured in this study. Nevertheless it is a well-conducted study showing the value of a fairly intense effort to reduce physician burnout and related matters. Physician burnout appears to affect over half of practicing physicians[52] so this is a serious matter concerning the clinical milieu for patients and physicians alike. The medical profession is a challenging occupation in the twenty-first century despite the riches of technological advancement and considerable financial remuneration. The physician is challenged from many directions including demanding patients, legal threats, authoritarian payers, intrusive bureaucracies, demanding accrediting organizations, and others. Instead of experiencing the independence of being the captain of a cottage industry as in the nineteenth and first half of the twentieth century when caring for the patient was relatively straightforward if arduous, and professionalism was maintained by both community and guild standards, physicians of the twenty-first century must answer to many bureaucratic stakeholders. A study of hospitals that had stress reduction programs for its employees including clinicians had a significant reduction in malpractice claims compared to comparable hospitals that did not have such programs.[53] Clearly other healthcare providers aside from physicians are subject to burnout and interventions can improve their patient interactions as well.

For some healthcare professionals today there is an element of exhaustion and dryness. It is reminiscent of when Gehlen described modern culture as "crystallized" wherein science and technology combine to devitalize societal institutions.[54] Habermas questioned this neo-conservative view of an exhaustion of cultural modernity but admits that technology and science does not provide as much guidance to the formation of lifeworlds and their related political and social institutions as earlier belief systems.[55] My point is that the overwhelming of the medical profession by a multitude of cultural changes, technological advancements and a plethora of powerful stakeholders can cause a desiccation of professionalism *per se*. If the postmodern medical lifeworld calls for diminished physician authority, more patient autonomy, increased bureaucratic control, and lessened professional satisfaction, those can be expected to have a non-salutary effect on the quality of medical care in the twenty-first century. The Levinasian Caring for the Other is constricted by a plethora of powerful stakeholders and their demands on clinicians.

A PLETHORA OF STAKEHOLDERS

The dominant voice of consumerism in our culture promotes individualism and self-interest because neither solidarity nor virtue is nourished in the marketplace. As Busch notes in his essay citing Adam Smith, dominant consumerism obliterates the social learning of virtue, so self-interest becomes a dominant feature.[56] Burnout ensues from a consumerist society stifling such things as beneficence, community, and altruism in conjunction with the incessant demands of multiple stakeholders, incessant advertising, and marketing.

Different stakeholders in healthcare also have a role in reshaping the medical professionalism of the twenty-first century. Of great interest now are the quality improvement initiatives that have been embraced by the payers of medical care such as CMS and private insurance companies as well as many other healthcare stakeholders. The Institute for Healthcare Improvement, a leading innovator in the quality improvement movement, was founded by the visionary Donald Berwick. The effort to contain costs had become linked to quality improvement with the notion that if complications are avoided costs will be reduced. Hence payers are increasingly interested and involved in the monitoring of quality. Good quality, while sometimes reducing costs, more often is costly and involves expensive technology.

The Joint Commission, the dominant accrediting agency of American hospitals is also a major effector of quality improvement initiatives. Their inspectors examine processes that promote quality improvement and set process standards for certification that are essential to hospital reimbursement by Federal agencies and other payers. It is a very important stakeholder in healthcare in the United States today.

Regarding the physician certification component, the member organizations of the American Board of Medical Specialties are demanding that physician board recertification require some measurement of quality in the physicians' actual practice of their medical specialty through process and outcomes measures. The respective medical specialty societies interact to varying degrees of effectiveness with the specialty boards. Patient stakeholders value courtesy, empathy, responsiveness, clinical effectiveness, and low out-of-pocket expense. Healthcare system executives value throughput efficiency, return on investment, marketable services, and strong operating margins. Physicians value recognition, ease of use, efficiency, financial reward, and good clinical outcomes. Nurses value respect, collaboration, responsiveness to their needs including working conditions as well as the needs of the patients and good clinical outcomes. Payers value return on investment, cost effective provision of services, marketability of services, and patient satisfaction. This multiplicity of stakeholders and their agendas make for a challenging, somewhat chaotic, medical milieu where most have concerns about their particular interests so that collaboration and trust are sometimes in short supply. There are some signs progress is being made in aligning these various objectives but much waits to be done in re-aligning incentives. A frank and accurate assessment of medical professionalism is essential to that progress. Expecting physicians to advocate for the primacy of patient interest over self-interest as has been touted[57] but is dated and unrealistic in view of how postmodern culture has developed in the late twentieth century and the early twenty-first century. Instead we can align enlightened self-interest with training methods that enhance empathy, reduce burnout, and improve emotional intelligence, as well as using advanced medical technology sensibly while respecting the needs of individuals and society at large. This will not be easy nor happen naturally in our culture but will take unprecedented effort and collaboration among the various stakeholders, intelligence both cognitive and emotional, courage, leadership, and a passion to improve the current state of affairs.

As Light notes "culture will shape what doctors do, how they feel and what is considered to be professional practice."[58] What is needed is the ability to understand where our culture has led and reestablish professional norms based on a realistic understanding of the new foundations of society and determine the standards of medical practice in the bedrock of postmodern culture. Once a bioethicist described my earlier communitarian views as obsolete in the late twentieth century, and I reluctantly now agree with her, although I do not subscribe to the radical individualism that often predominates in a consumerist-oriented society. Instead one should encourage all medical stakeholders to embrace the best of postmodern culture rather than mourn the demise of values of an earlier era. New types of training methodologies could improve how physicians communicate with their patients and feel about their work. In this way we may be able to replace the best of intentions with best practices that improve the experience of healthcare as well as its outcomes. One cannot retreat to prior values but one can plan, do, study and act[59] to improve the *status quo* ethically as well as technically. We need to collaborate across disciplines and stakeholders to revitalize medical professionalism with a new awareness of the changed moral milieu of the twenty-first century.

NOTES

1. Osler W. *Aequanimitas: With other addresses to medical students.* 2nd ed. Philadelphia: Blakiston's Son, 1920) p. 386.

2. King M. L. Jr., http://www.brainyquote.com/quotes/quotes/m/martinluth132188.html. Accessed June 12, 2013.

3. Parsons T. *The Social System.* Routledge Kegan Paul, London, 1951.

4. Bliss Michael. *Osler: A Life in Medicine.* New York: Oxford Univ Press. 1999.

5. Lantos J. RVUs blues. How should docs get paid? *Hastings Center Report* 33(3):37–45, 2003.

6. Jessup M. Truth the First Casualty of Postmodern Consumerism. *Christian Scholar's Review* 2001; 30(3)289–304.

7. Lyotard, J.-F., 1984, *The Postmodern Condition: A Report on Knowledge*, Geoff Bennington and Brian Massumi (trans.), Minneapolis: University of Minnesota Press.

8. Marcus Welby, MD. http://en.wikipedia.org/wiki/Marcus_Welby,_M.D..

9. Ginzberg E. The Monetarization of Medical Care. *N Engl J Med* 1984; 210(18) p. 1163.

10. Angell M. Big Pharma, Bad Medicine. *Boston Review.* May/June 2010 http://bostonreview.net/BR35.3/angell.php. accessed November 11, 2012.

11. Smith R. Medical journals are an extension of the market arm of pharmaceutical companies. *PLoS Med.* 2005 May; 2 (5) : e138.

12. Safe Surgery Saves Lives. http://www.who.int/patientsafety/safesurgery/en/. Accessed November 11, 2012.

13. Patient Like Me Blog. http://blog.patientslikeme.com/ Accessed December 11, 2012.

14. Illingworth P. Trust: the scarcest of medical resources. *J Med Phil* 2002; 27(1): 31–46.

15. Gerber B. S., Eiser A. R. The patient-physician relationship in the Internet Age: Future prospects and the research agenda. *J Med Internet Research* 2001; 3(2): e15.

16. Chaitlin E., Stiller R., Jacobs S., et al. Physician—patient relationship in the intensive care unit: Erosion of sacred trust? *Crit Care Med* 2003; 31(5)suppl S367–S372.

17. Safran D. G., Taira D. A., Rogers W. H., et al. Linking primary care performance to outcomes of care. *J Fam Med* 1998; 47: 213–20.

18. Federation of State Medical Boards Summary of Actions 2009. http://www.fsmb.org/pdf/2009-summary-board-actions.pdf.

19. Cruess S. R., Johnston S., Cruess R. L. Professionalism for Medicine: Opportunities and Obligations. *Med J Aus* 2002; 177:208–211.

20. Kearney R. A. Defining professionalism in anesthesiology. *Medical Education* 2005; 39:769–776.

21. Hafferty F. W. What medical students know about professionalism. *Mt. Sinai J Med* 2002; 69:385–397.

22. Gillespie C., Palik S., Ark T., et al. Resident perception of their own professionalism and the professionalism of their learning environment. *J Grad Med Education* 2009; 1: 208–215.

23. Bishop J. P., Rees C. E. Hero or has-been: is there a future for altruism in medical education? *Ad Health Sci Educ Theory Prac* 2007: 12:391–399.

24. Hamilton, W. D., 1975, Innate Social Aptitudes in Man: an Approach from Evolutionary Genetics, in *Biosocial Anthropology*, R. Fox (ed.), New York: Wiley.

25. Jones R. Declining altruism in medicine. *Br Med J* 2002; 324:625–626.

26. Barber B. *Strong Democracy* Berkeley, 1984. Pp. 17–18.

27. Ci J. Disenchantment, desublimation, demoralization: some cultural conjunctions of capitalism. *New Literary History* 1999, 30(2):295–324.

28. Lipton D. Consumerism, reflexivity, and the medical encounter. *Soc Sci Med* 1997; 45(3): 373–381.

29. Lyotard, J.-F., 1984, *The Postmodern Condition: A Report on Knowledge*, Geoff Bennington and Brian Massumi (trans.), Minneapolis: University of Minnesota Press.

30. Brame R. G. What happened to altruism. *Obst Gyn* 2008; 112(3):687–688.

31. Franan J. M., Paro J. A., Higa J., et al. The YouTube Generation: implications for medical professionalism. *Perspective Bio Med* 2008; 51(4):517–524.

32. Burbules N. C. Postmodern doubt and the philosophy of education. http://www.ed.uiuc.edu/eps/PES/95_dpcs/burbules,html.

33. MacCann C., Roberts R. D. New paradigm for assessing emotional intelligence. *Emotion* 2008; 8(4):540–551.

34. Daniel Goleman. *Emotional Intelligence: Why It Can Matter More Than IQ*. New York: Bantam 1997.

35. Druskat V. U., Sala F., Mount G. *Linking Emotional Intelligence and performance at work: Current research evidence with individuals and groups*. Erlbaum, Mahwash NJ 2006.

36. Stratton T. D., Elam C. L., Murphy-Spencer A. E., Qunilivan S. L. Emotional Intelligence and clinical skills: preliminary results forma a comprehensive clinical performance examination. *Acad Med* 2005; 80(10suppl) S34–S37.

37. Carrothers R. M., Gregory S. W., Gallagher T. J. Measuring emotional intelligence of medical school matriculants. *Acad Med* 75:456–463, 2000.

38. Wagner P., Ginger M. X., Grant M. M., et al. Physicians' emotional intelligence and patient satisfaction. *Fam Med* 2002; 34:750–754.

39. Chen D., Lew R., Hershman W., Orlander J. A cross-sectional measurement of medical student empathy. *JGIM* 2007;22(10):434–438.

40. Kim S. S., Kaplowitz S., Johnston M. V. The effect of physician empathy on patient satisfaction and compliance. *Eval Health Prof* 2004; 27:237–241.

41. Mangione S., Kane G. C., Caruso J. W., et al. Assessment of empathy in different years if internal medicine training. *Medical Teacher* 24(4):370-373, 2002.

42. Ludwig D. S., Kabat-Zinn J. Mindfulness in Medicine. *JAMA* 2008; 300(11):1350–1352.

43. Winston K. Atheism rises, religiondeclines.http://www.huffingtonpost.com/2012/08/14/atheism-rise-religiosity-decline-in-america_n_1777031.html. Accessed June 20, 2013.

44. Allen D., Wainwright M., Mount B. M., Hutchinson T. The wounding path to becoming healers. *Med Teach* 2008; 30(3):260–264.

45. Hutchinson T. A., Dobkin P. L. Mindful medical practice: Just another fad? *Canad Fam Physician* 2009; 55:778–779.

46. Kabat-Zinn J. *Full Catastrophe living: Using the wisdom of your body and mind to face stress, pain, and illness*, New York, NY: Dell Publishing; 1990.

47. Lutz A., Brefczynski-Lewis J. A., Johnstone T., Davidson R. J. Voluntary Regulation of Neural Circuitry of Emotion by Compassion Meditation: Effects of Expertise. *PLOS One* 3:e1897, 2008.

48. Ambady N., LaPlante D., Nguyen T., et al. Surgical Tone of Voice. *Surgery* 2002; 132:5–9.

49. Hickson G. B., Federspiel C. F., Pichert J. W., Miller C. S. Patient complaints and malpractice risk. *JAMA* 2002; 287:2951–7.

50. Billier-Amdorno N., Lee T. H. Ethical Incentives-From Carrots and Sticks. *N Engl J Med* 368(11):980–982, 2013.

51. Krasner M. S., Epstein R. M., Beckman H., Suchman A. L., et al. Association an education program in mindful communication with burnout, empathy, attitudes among primary care physicians. *JAMA* 2009; 302(12):1284–1293.

52. Spickard A. Jr., Gabbe S. G., Christensen J. F. Mid-career burnout in generalist and specialist physicians. *JAMA* 2002; 288(12):1447–1450.

53. Jones J. W., Barge B. N., Steffy B. D., Fay L. M., Kunz L. K., Weubker L. J. Stress and medical malpractice: organization risk assessment and intervention. *J Appl Psychol.* 1988; 73(4):727–735.

54. A. Gehlen. Uber kulturelle Kristalizatkion. In *Studien zur Anthropologie and Soziologie Neuwied*, 1963, p. 321.

55. Habermas J. Neoconservative Cutural Criticism in the United States and West Germany: An Intellectual Movement in Two Political Cultures. In *Habermas and Modernity* edit. Bernstein R. J. Polity Press 1985. Part 1 Chapter 3.

56. Busch M. Adam Smith and consumerism's role in happiness: Modern society re-examined. *Major Themes in Economics*. Spring 2008 65–77.

57. Stern D. T., Papadakis M. The developing physician—becoming a professional. *N Engl J Med* 2006; 355:1794–1749.

58. Light D. W. Countervailing powers, a framework for professions in transition. In Johnson T., Larkin G., Saks M., eds. *Healthcare Professions and the State in Europe*. London: Roultedge. 1995; 25–41.

59. Plan Do Study Act. Institute for Healthcare Improvement. http://www.ihi.org/knowledge/Pages/Tools/PlanDoStudyActWorksheet.aspx. Accessed December 11, 2012.

Chapter Nine

The Postmodern Physician Ethos and Morale

"We know that every profession is in danger of collapsing when another end is imposed upon it . . . even if it is initially only appended to it." —Jean-Francois Lyotard[1]

"The first task of the doctor is . . . political: the struggle against disease must begin with a war against bad government. Man will be totally and definitively cured only if he is first liberated. . ." —Michel Foucault[2]

PHYSICIAN MORALE: A GLOBAL MALAISE

I wrote this chapter in the wake of the 2012 triple disaster in Japan; earthquake, tsunami, and nuclear reactor failure. Frightening as this catastrophe was, I was equally startled to discover another type of Japanese disaster described in a 2008 article entitled "The Catastrophic Collapse of Morale among Hospital Physicians in Japan" by Hideo Yasunaga, a healthcare management professor.[3] The article describes poor morale arising from overwork, patients' adversarial view of physicians, poor reimbursement, physician shortages, hostile depiction of physicians in the media, mounting malpractice suits (in a country usually not litigious), and verbal and physical abuse of physicians and other healthcare providers. A study of nearly 500 physicians indicated that 29 percent had experienced physical violence or abusive language from patients in the prior six months.[4] Gone is the veneration of physicians, as in a bygone era, replaced by a consumerist model characterized by high expectations of flawless and speedy clinical services on demand from limited and strained physician resources. Physician *karoshi* (death by overwork) and *karojisatsu* (suicide by overwork) have been documented in the Japanese occupational medicine literature.[5] "Catastrophic collapse of physician morale" should raise very serious concern, and it is by no means confined to Japan. For one thing it is hard to get peak or even par performances from professionals with low morale who feel trapped by their professional circumstances in a hostile setting of bureaucratic and patient demands. Besides, physicians at their best demand a great deal of themselves. In addition, it is difficult to attract new talent to a profession if it is embroiled in turmoil. Students in today's elite undergraduate colleges may consider a career in medicine as sacrificing the best years of their young adulthood to a "thankless job" with undesirable work/life balance and a questionable return on their investment of time, effort, and money.

As Zygmunt Bauman has cogently observed, "postmodern living means living with strangers, and living with strangers is at times a precarious, unnerving and testing life."[6] The estrangement at the bedside or in the clinic is part and parcel of a larger cultural milieu. Media coverage of medical errors and other physician misdeeds, Internet-based information available to patients including patient blogs, physician ratings, and medical information have drastically changed patients' perceptions of physicians and physicians' perceptions of their own position in society. The medical bureaucracies including health insurers and healthcare provider systems challenge patient and physician alike in a clinical encounter that is highly technology-focused including the use of electronic medical records and imaging technology, as well as advanced invasive therapies, including monoclonal antibodies targeting specific cell functions and robotic surgery. Information technology has forever changed the clinical encounter. However, even in simple clinical encounters, the physician may feel the social forces of a consumerist ethos reduce her authority and sense of accomplishment. Reading a physician blog concerning emergency department (ED) physicians, I noticed a complaint that ED physicians in the United States may receive calls from hospital administrators recommending the ED physicians should be less reluctant to prescribe narcotic pain relievers when the patients request them.[7] Because of a federal government mandate for a particular patient satisfaction survey known as the HCAHPS survey whereby patients indicate, among other questions, whether they received adequate pain relief. A low score on the HCAHPS survey may discourage Internet savvy patients from utilizing that particular ED. Hence the consumerist model of medical care reduces the physician to a technocrat subject to market-driven pressures. Morris notes that pain in the postmodern era has *grown* exponentially to epidemic proportions and that the biomedical model fails to account for this growth.[8] He further mentions that the distinctively postmodern developments includes class action litigation and politically influential patient organizations. So physicians, at times, may feel hapless in such circumstances when consumerist forces dominate either their decision-making or that of healthcare executives. As the Lyotard quote at the beginning of this chapter observes, appending such roles to the physician role as keeping the consumer happy may have untoward negative impact on the profession going so far as to deprofessionalize it to some extent. In addition, the corporate commercial model undermines the promise in the Hippocratic tradition of physicians to care for the sick regardless of socioeconomic status.[9] So two elements in the postmodern proposition, consumerist and corporate, engender lower morale of physicians and lessening of medical professionalism. Durante called attention to the "physician's fragility" in addition to the patient's fragility, and observed that legalistic influences in clinical medicine can adversely impact both parties in the clinical encounter.[10]

A survey of over 1,200 American physicians, published in *Physician Executive* in 2006, notes that over 60 percent have considered leaving the practice of medicine.[11] Causes of low morale include declining reimbursement, loss of autonomy, bureaucratic administrative "red tape," patient overload, loss of respect by patients, and the malpractice environment. Emotional burnout was reported by over two-thirds, depression and marital discord by roughly a third of physicians, and suicidal thoughts by over 4 percent. The pain and discomfort of clinical practice are not distributed equally in all specialties. General internal medicine had the lowest satisfaction score and the highest burnout scores in a survey of Kaiser Permanente physicians.[12] Primary care physicians experience a disproportionate amount of the bureaucratic minutiae of clinical practice regarding certifying consults, imaging studies, and other evaluations and clinical services when the insured services are highly controlled. However, all types of physicians are experiencing bureaucratic intrusion to varying degrees. Other clinicians including nurses[13] and nurse practitioners are feeling similar. Over half the nurses in this Canadian study reported severe burnout.

How does postmodern culture contribute to physician low morale? Loss of autonomy is attributable to corporate takeover of the delivery of medical care in the era of late capitalism, and the growth of regulatory bureaucracies and exponential growth of requirements. The growing demands on physicians' time and effort are impacted as more of the human condition is medicalized, more preventive measures are identified and entered into guidelines, more discrete clinical data entry is required, and more arduous re-certification procedures are required. The postmodern exponential growth of scientific and technological information, and the computerization of the medical information and administrative processes creates a sense of information overload. Such overload also contributes to burnout.

The declining status of physicians in the popular culture also contributes to a sense of burnout. Loss of respect arises from media and press coverage of physician misconduct, loss of community sensibility, multi-cultural and cross-cultural miscommunication, moral relativism, and other postmodern cultural phenomena. Lyotard has noted in the *Postmodern Condition* that computerized communications have contributed to the loss of grand narratives in society and the public sphere.[14] More online reports of physicians' misdeeds fuel a diminution of respect for physicians, which in turn makes the tasks of the physician more difficult to accomplish as respect and trust are vital to clinical effectiveness.

The medical liability environment is intensified by these postmodern developments that include the extensive advertising of law firms, both online and through other electronic media.[15] Patients are angry because of poor outcomes, poor communication, brusqueness and aloofness of physicians, financial pressures, and long waits for treatment.[16] The mere specter of a medical liability suit can haunted a physician.

Sleep deprivation of physicians from constant electronic media bombardment and computerized data heighten tension in the clinical encounter. Some are uniquely related to postmodern uses of electronic media especially with the LCD screens delaying bedtime and shortening total sleep time.[17] Sleep deprivation is known to make people irritable and antagonistic. So the postmodern clinical encounter is likely to involve both parties who are somewhat sleep deprived and not likely to be focused on Levinas' Face of the Other, adding to both parties' displeasure. There is a large body of literature about the influence of fatigue on resident physicians and their clinical performance as well as many policy regulatory changes by the ACGME[18] but very little on sleep deprivation of the patient or the attending physician in postmodern culture which is part of a much larger picture of sleep disturbances in the United States and other countries.

Physician burnout has been reported from a wide variety of nations: Japan, China, United States, Canada, United Kingdom, Germany, The Netherlands, Finland, Herzegovina, and others. In Canada, general practitioners are retiring and new ones are not taking their places; over 2 million Quebecois citizens lack a family physician due to the severe shortage.[19] Trying to provide care in this primary care discipline is frustrating and poorly remunerated compared to specialties. There may be little sense of accomplishment as a primary care physician if one is often spending time completing forms for specialty referrals that the patients insist upon even if the generalist physician can handle the problem. All consumers want the best clinical services for themselves, and many assume the specialist assures the best outcome for them. While that is often the case, there are times when it is not simply not so.

One does not need to wait until practicing as an attending physician to experience a sense of burnout. Resident physicians and medical students also score highly on burnout measures. Thirty percent of Dutch medical residents met the criteria of burnout on the Maslach inventory.[20] Psychiatric residents experienced the most emotional exhaustion in that study. Practicing physicians in the United Kingdom report that their professionalism is belittled by decreased time with patients because of the increased amount of time and effort in revalidating their credentials that now include an annual performance review.[21] Medical students in Minnesota report a 45 percent burnout rate leading to and developing a tendency "to treat people as less than human and more as objects."[22] Burnout included emotional exhaustion, depersonalization, and low sense of personal accomplishment. Over 55 percent of medical students scored positive on a screen for depression. The number of negative personal life events correlated with the risk of burnout. Being a medical student provides no immunity to the stresses of postmodern life. Depersonalization is the subset of burnout that has been shown to correlate with poor professionalism behavior.[23] Depersonalization is also, not surprisingly, associated with lower patient satisfaction and longer post-discharge recovery time;[24] in other words worse patient outcomes. Burnout begets lower patient satisfaction as the physician also experiences dissatisfaction. In pre-postmodern times, the myth of the physician did, to some extent, "immunize" medical students, resident physicians, and attending physicians from life stresses as we believed in the myth of the larger-than-life physician.

So the unfolding story of physician morale globally is one of mutual distress. Is this a uniquely postmodern phenomenon? Medical training has always been stressful. In the past the hours were longer, the pay was less, supervision less rigorous, and the ACGME did not exist to help protect trainees from excesses of their teachers, real and imagined. So why should burnout be so much greater now? Physicians were once highly regarded in the society, were expected to make great personal sacrifice, but also were expected to occupy a position that was honored and rewarded both financially and emotionally. The loss of grand narratives that so characterizes the postmodern era has impacted the most those who had the greatest distance to fall, and medical professionals are certainly among them. The heroic status once conferred actually was a major factor in buffering the psyche of someone who chose the healing professions. The loss of status of the health professional reverberates through the clinical encounter and adversely affects patients as well as the physicians themselves. The social forces that wrought these changes include the extensive media coverage of medicine's faults, electronic communication, loss of community, moral relativism, consumerist ideology, corporate control of medical practice, and the multiculturalism ethos of postmodern life. Unintended consequences of postmodernism impact all aspects of modern life including the complex social-technological nexus of healthcare. Postmodernism tends to be interpreted as denying the existence of cultural universals but in this instance it appears that postmodernism is creating a new cultural universal: *physician burnout*. A study in Poland helps elucidate one of the mechanisms for this disenchantment. It shows that patient non-compliance is a major factor. In a study of how physicians respond to patient non-compliance to the medical regimen, Heszen-Klemens found that patient non-compliance is perceived as an ego-threatening event by the majority of physicians which is accompanied by strong negative emotions.[25] The author notes that patients are similarly experiencing frustration as both the disease and its treatment are infringing on their life goals and lifestyle. But from the physician perspective, a patient declining to follow the prescribed regimen is offensive. In the new Pay for Performance processes being implemented by American insurers and CMS, patient non-compliance could also adversely affect the physicians' ratings and bonus payments as non-compliance reduces quality measures of process and/or outcome.[26] Pay for Performance has become prominent as a way to assure compliance with practice guidelines. Patients' options not to comply have always existed but now they take on additional meaning for the clinician as internal and external bureaucracies will be making their own measurement of clinical processes and clinical outcomes.

Patient non-compliance is estimated to contribute to 125,000 deaths per year and add $150 billion to the cost of medical care in the United States.[27] Thus non-compliance does considerably more than merely aggravate physicians; it is injurious to the patients themselves. While it may be obvious, I think it is helpful to note that both physicians and patients live and interact in the postmodern social and moral milieu of a fast paced "liquid modern" world that devalues duration and hierarchy, where information obliterates narrative,[28] and a substantial number of individuals are anxious, demanding, and impatient. The egalitarian attitude of the consumerist perspective does not necessarily mean that either party, patient or physician, will be pleased with the encounter. A vague unease may permeate the interaction where uncertainty of roles, attitudes, and responsibilities characterize the postmodern clinical encounter. The Patient-Physician Agreement that I described in an earlier chapter may help in this regard if it were to be implemented. Neither patients nor physicians are likely to be compliant with guidelines unless both have some "skin in the game," personal investment in the healing process. Perhaps we need to consider letting patients share in the payoff when benchmarks are met, at least to some extent.

POSTMODERN PHYSICIAN MISCONDUCT

The flip side of low physician morale is physician misconduct in the clinical arena. As I noted above, low morale is related to living in a milieu of exponential growth of electronic information, loss of the physicians status as Foucault had described it in an earlier era, "sovereign as the questioner, the observing eye, touching finger. . ."[29] loss of control of practice to corporations, certifying organizations, credentialing and monitoring processes, intentions to have work/life balance, and the general uncertainty of "liquid" post-modern life. Could these same influences account for physician misconduct? Possibly, but it is probably more complex than that.

Physician misconduct may take several forms but that most commonly mentioned is what is termed by the Joint Commission (on Hospital and Healthcare organizations accreditation) disruptive physicians. This usually refers to threatening or abusive language, condescending language, even threat of physical abuse, and sometimes, physical abuse.[30] The physicians likely to engage in this misconduct are more often surgeons both general and surgical specialists (75 percent) although cardiologists and gastroenterologists also make the list.[31] This also suggests that the social ethos is different for highly paid proceduralists that generate large hospital revenues as well as large professional fees, and have had an even longer period of post-graduate medical training (six to nine years instead of three years for primary care specialties). It may attract a more aggressive, ambitious, and demanding individuals who can perform complicated invasive procedures under considerable stress and duress. So while misconduct may involve primary care physicians, the focus of disruptive physicians is more the specialists who perform complicated procedures. Surgeons are also accustomed to rising early in the morning (5 am) and commonly experience fatigue and sleep deprivation both during training and for their entire professional lives. Sleep deprivation and the ensuing fatigue may contribute to their irritability in the operating suite but should not justify misbehavior there or elsewhere. Some surgeons will cancel scheduled surgeries if they have a nocturnal emergency case but many will not.[32] So the pace of postmodern liquid life with its hurried pace, high expectations (no cancellations), high pressure social and economic environment may at least in part account for some instances of misconduct. Also the unique challenges in the operating suite (OS) include the challenge of arousing the other members of the team from their routines to suddenly deal with the crises that can develop very acutely during surgical procedures. This is not a uniquely postmodern problem but postmodern changes in attitudes and expectations may intensify the tension in the OS. Although new quality improvement initiatives like the checklists have been shown to improve patient safety, some surgeons may view them as encroaching on their authority.

Bauman offers several insights that contribute to understanding what is happening in the clinical encounter. He notes that the moral self cannot survive the fragmentation of social and professional life that is engendered by advancing technology.[33] He further states that technological advancement leads to an increasing volume and intensity of systemic imbalances. He quotes Jacques Ellul, "What counts is the convergence on man of a plurality . . . of systems or complexes of techniques. The result is operational totalitarianism; no longer is any part of man free and independent of these techniques."[34] So both physician and patient in the clinical encounter are captured by a complex of techniques experienced in clinical practice that *operates* on both the physician and the patient. Corporate influences range from the healthcare system, the multi-specialty group practice management, the product manufacturers, the insurers, the accrediting agencies, the quality improvement organizations, and the medical liability legal interests. The moral self that should be at the fore of medical practice is submerged in the morass of multiple stakeholder interests, many seeking to expand their role and influence. All are driving the moral aspects of medicine to the margins of the processes.

PHYSICIAN-NURSING DISJUNCTIONS

Rosenstein and O'Daniel studied disruptive behavior in the operating suite (OS) and found while surgeons were the greatest offenders they were followed closely by anesthesiologists, and in descending frequency by OS nurses, surgical and anesthesia residents, surgical technicians, and CRNAs.[35] They note that disruptive behavior can have significant adverse effect on patient outcomes. They recommend the implementation of formal rules for communicating issues, the teaching of team dynamics and communication skills, and designating teamwork champions among the physician and nursing ranks. The Joint Commission is calling on hospitals to demonstrate how they deal with disruptive healthcare professionals.[36] But physicians counter that administrators may try to use this policy to remove physicians with opinions differing from their own. Nursing perspectives are substantially different and express the need to confront physicians who ignore safety checklists as reported by the Association of periOperative Registered Nurses (AORN). Disruptive physician behavior is a frequently-cited reason given by nurses for voluntarily leaving a hospital.[37] A survey of physician executives notes that the most common type of disruptive physician behaviors are being disrespectful of nurses and, less often, exhibiting similar behavior toward patients or administrators.[38] The authors of this study cite contributing factors such as physician-nurse antagonism, physician refusal to embrace a team approach, and physician frustration at organizational changes in medical practice. The last factor can be seen as a postmodern development: the corporate control of the practice of medicine. Physician-nurse antagonism could be viewed as a battle within the postmodern flattened hierarchy embraced by nurses and more enlightened physicians but fiercely resisted by a minority of physicians who may not change unless an effective intervention occurs. The intervention may not occur if the administration fears that the physician will take his patients and procedures elsewhere. Physicians and administrators are also impacted by increased regulatory requirements, lower reimbursements, and a reluctance to acknowledge the cultural changes that nurses have embraced in raising their professional consciousness. The postmodern organization is characterized by ambiguity and shifting power relationships. Lyotard writes of the ambiguous postmodern evolution of social interactions, be they professional, emotional, gender-based, cultural, or political. [39] In the case of the nurse-physician interaction all those factors are combined in a complex nexus of frustrated interactions that can be potentially dissatisfying. Change, particularly ambiguous change, is anxiety provoking and stressful. Today's healthcare organizations must recognize a multiplicity of stakeholders and attempt to balance competing needs, values, opinions, and ideologies. This is a daunting but necessary task. The current state is imperfect in its applications because it is difficult to satisfy disparate, contrasting values, ideologies, and needs. In a later chapter I will suggest some approaches that appear to be working in creating more accord and less disruptive behavior. Right now the tsunami of social change has churned up strong emotions in physicians, nurses, and administrators alike and all parties are feeling some discomfort.

Several studies have found that as a group, physicians have low emotional intelligence; one found that in a sample of Canadian and American physicians their emotional intelligence quotient was below average. [40] A study in the United States found EQ declining during medical school. [41] Another study found a decline in empathy during residency training. [42] I would suggest that low EQ starts before medical school in medical students and declines during training, and that this contributes to both low morale and physician misconduct. The practice of medicine has always been difficult but never more so in postmodern times while medical students are selected by cognitive intelligence not emotional intelligence.

A study in Slovenia indicates that both nurses and physicians felt a low level of personal involvement in their work, and low employment satisfaction because of the imposition of a hierarchical organizational culture where neither profession felt they could display their professional integrity. [43] So both physician morale and nurse morale influence one another, but the corporate influence over medical practice and the values it imputes to the clinical encounter including standardization and disempowerment of medical professionals may be the greatest changing influence and contributor to low morale.

Moral relativism arising from the multiplicity and complexity of social values in postmodern society constricts physicians' values as well as those of other citizens. As Bauman has stated, "the moral self is the most evident and the most prominent among technology's victims." [44] This does not justify physician misconduct but it does help to explains its origin and causes. It also suggests that merely exhorting physicians to return to the moral order of the nineteenth and early-twentieth centuries is not likely to succeed. There is a need to develop post-postmodern epistemes that can counter the consumerist, corporate, individualistic, and materialistic epistemes of postmodern culture. If these new epistemes can engender a new model of concern for the Other then a renewed ethos may replace and replenish the current dispirited one. One can conceive of a countervailing social force that expresses care of the Other, and related humanizing values, but these are not currently operative or apparent at the current moment in medical history. These new epistemes should foster an environment wherein physicians and nurses are more willing to work in collaborative teams. The patient also should become more of a willing participant in their own care, rather than strictly a consumer of healthcare. This will require a considerable re-imagining and restructuring of medical care to incorporate some communitarian values rather than permit the business consumerist ethos to dominate disproportionately as it does today.

SUMMARY OF POSTMODERN INFLUENCES ON PHYSICIAN MORALE AND MISCONDUCT

The loss of the grand myth of the physician and the flattening of the medical hierarchy has constituted a significant blow to physician morale. Back in the days when resident physicians worked 90–100 hours per week, we were "immunized" from that hardship and privation by the thought that we were, in some regard, special. Physician low EQ may not be a new phenomenon but it has certainly become more apparent with the demise of the cultural myth of the physician. The technological juggernaut of computerization of medical information and the increased corporate oversight of medical practice through financial and quality management adds exponentially to the complexity and stress of medical practice. The stress and fatigue of postmodern life are further exacerbated by all the electronic accoutrements and the exponential growth of information. The postmodern corporate influences engender *anomie*, power dislocation, and financial aggrandizement. Powerful pharmaceutical companies, device manufacturers, healthcare delivery systems, health insurance companies, and accrediting healthcare and professional organizations directly and indirectly influence the medical cultural ethos within which physicians and nurses pursue their professions to care for patients.

There is a need to think more imaginatively in creating new medical epistemes. They will need to draw upon advances in neurosciences, psychology, and neuroethics as well as older, established techniques for developing teambuilding, fostering greater mindfulness in clinical practice, and engendering greater emotional intelligence in the clinical setting. I am suggesting an ambitious project to create a post-postmodern ethos for a more robust and humane moral setting for medical practice.

NOTES

1. Lyotard Jean-Francois. *The Postmodern Explained*. Minneapolis: Univ. of Minnesota Press, 1993.

2. Foucault M. *The Birth of the Clinic*. London: Routledge 1989, p. 38. http://www.goodreads.com/author/quotes/1260.Michel_Foucault.

3. Yasunaga H. The catastrophic collapse of morale among hospital physicians in Japan. *Risk Management and Healthcare Policy* 1:1–6, 2008.

4. Wada K., Yoshida K., Sato E. The situation of patient violence and the measurement of it. *Nihon Iji Shinpo* 4354:81–84, 2007.

5. Hiyama T., Yoshihara M. New Occupational threats to Japanese physicians: karoshi (death by overwork) and karojisatsu (suicide by overwork). *Occupation Environ Med* 65:428–429, 2008.

6. Bauman Z. *Liquid Modernity*. Cambridge, UK: Polity, 2000. P. 91.

7. Leap E. How Patient Satisfaction can Affect Physicians. http://www.kevinmd.com/blog/2010/02/patient-satisfaction-scores-affect-physicians.html. Accessed July 7, 2011.

8. Morris David B., *Reinventing Pain in Illness and Culture in the Postmodern Age*. Berkeley: Univ California Press, 1998, p. 107–134.

9. Hiu E. C. The contractual model of the patient-physician relationship and the demise of medical professionalism. *Hong Kong Medicine* 1(5): 420–422, 2005.

10. Durante C. The Physician's Frailty. *AJOB* 9(10): 33–35, 2009.

11. Steiger B. Survey Results: Doctors Say Morale is Hurting. *Physician Executive* 11: Nov–Dec 2006, 6–15.

12. Freeborn, D. Satisfaction, commitment and psychological well-being among HMO physicians. *Western J Medicine*, 174, 13–1, 2001.

13. Greco P., Spence Lashinger H. K., Wong C. Leadership Empowering Behaviours, Staff Nurse Empowerment and Work Engage/Burnout. *Nursing Research* 19(4):41–43, 2006.

14. Grant, Iain H. *Postmodernism and Science and Technology*, in *The Routledge Companion to Postmodernism*. London: Routledge, 2005, p. 66.

15. Vukmir R. B. Medical Malpractice: Managing the Risk. *Medicine & Law* 33:495–513, 2004.

16. Murtagh J. The Angry Patient. *Australian Family Physician* 20(4):388–389, 1991.

17. Cain N., Gradisar M. Electronic media and sleep deprivation in children and students. *Sleep Medicine* 11(8): 735–742, 2010.

18. Sen S., Kranzler H. R., Didwania A. K., et al. Effects of Duty Hours Reforms on Interns and their Patients. *JAMA Intern Med* 2013 1-6. doi:10.1001/jama internmed.2013.351.

19. Gore B. Shortage of Family Physicians in Quebec. *Montreal Gazette*. July 9, 2006. http://www.lexis.nexis.com.ezproxy2.library.drexel.edu/lnacui2api/delivery/PrintDoc.do"kp. Accessed March 21, 2011.

20. Prins J. T., Hoekstra J. E. H. M., van de Wiel H. B. M., et al. Burnout among Dutch medical residents. *Int J Behavioral Med* 14(3): 119–125, 2007.

21. PR Newswire August 6, 2008. UK Physicians fear new revalidation procedures will reduce morale, decrease time with patients and belittle GP professionalism, according to new TNS Healthcare Research. http://www.lexisnexis.com/ezproxy2.library. Accessed 3/16/11.

22. Dyrbye L. N., Thomas M. R., Huntington J. L., et al. Personal life events and medical student burnout: A multicenter study. *Acad Medicine* 81: 374–384, 2006.

23. Shanafelt T. D., Bradley K. A., Wipf J. E., Back A. L. Burnout and self-reported patient care in an internal medicine residency program. *Ann Intern Med* 36: 358–367, 2002.

24. Halbesieben J. R., Rathert C. Linking physician burnout and patient outcomes; exploring the dyadic relationship between physicians and patients. *Health Care Manage Rev* 33(1):29–39, 2008.

25. Heszen-Klemens I. Patient Noncompliance and How Doctors Manage This. *Soc Sci Med* 24(5):409–419, 1987.

26. Rosenthal M. B., Dudley R. A. Pay-for-performance: Will the latest payment trend improve care? *JAMA* 297:740–4, 2007.

27. Prange S. Improving Home Healthcare Through Telemedicine. http://ezinearticles.com/?Improving-Home-Healthcare-Through.

28. Zygmunt B. *Does Ethics Have A Chance in a World of Consumers?* Cambridge, MA: Harvard Univ Press, 2008.

29. Foucault M. *The Archeology of Knowledge and the Discourse of Language*. Trans. AM Sheridan Smith. New York: Pantheon, 1972, p. 53.

30. O'Reilly K. B. New Joint Commission standard tells hospitals to squelch disruptive behaviors. *American Medical News*. August 18, 2008.

31. Rosenstein A. H., O'Daniel M. Managing disruptive physicians' behavior: Impact on staff relationships and patient care. *Neurology* April 22, 2008, 70: 1564–1570.

32. Neuric M., Czeisler C. A. Sleep Deprivation, Elective Surgery, Informed Consent. *N Engl J Med* 2010; 363:2577–2579, 2010.

33. Zygmunt B. *Postmodern Ethics*. Oxford: Blackwell. 1993, p. 198.

34. Ellul J. *The Technological Society*. New York: Alfred A. Knopf, 1964, 389–391.

35. Rosenstein A. H., O'Daniel M. Impact and Implications of Disruptive Behavior in the Perioperative Arena. *J Am Col Surg* 203(1):96–105, 2006.

36. O'Reilly K. AMA News 8/18/08 Joint Commission standard tells hospitals to squelch disruptive behavior.

37. Sandrick K. Disruptive Physicians: an old problem comes under new scrutiny in an era of patient safety. *Trustee* November-December 2009, 2–12.

38. Weber D. O. Poll Results: Doctors' Disruptive Behavior Disturbs Physician Leaders. *Physician Executive*. Sept–Oct 2004, 4–14.

39. Lyotard J.-F. *The Postmodern Condition: A Report on Knowledge*. Transl. Geoff Bennington B. Massumi. Minneapolis: Univ Minnesota Press. 1979, p. 66.

40. Swift D. Do Doctors have an Emotional Handicap? *Medical Post* 35.10 March 9, 1999, 30.

41. Wagner P. J., Jester D. N., Albrittion T. A., Fincher R. M., Moseley C. M. Emotional Intelligence changes during medical school. *Teach Learn Med* 17(4):391–395, 2005.

42. Bellini L. M., Shea J. M. Mood change and empathy decline persist during three years of internal medicine training. *Acad Med* 80:164–167, 2005.

43. Savic B. S., Pagon M. Relationship between Nurses and Physicians in Terms of Organization Culture: Who is Responsible for Subordination of Nurses? *Croatian Med J* 49:334–343, 2008.

44. Bauman Z. *Postmodern Ethics*. Oxford: Blackwell, 198.

Chapter Ten

Bioethics in Postmodern America

"To save a man's life against his will is the same as killing him." —Horace
(Quintus Horatius Flaccus)[1]

"Postmodernism vitiates human rights to the extent it erects itself on the lack
of relation to the realities of the subordinated." —Catharine MacKinnon[2]

". . . a postmodern ethics would be one that readmits the Other as a neighbor,
as the close to hand—*and*—mind, into the hardcore of the moral self, back
from the wasteland of calculated interests to which it had been exiled."
—Zygmunt Bauman[3]

BIOETHICS AND THE END OF PATERNALISM

Contemporary bioethics became established by the 1960s, led first by theolo-
gians, and then by secular philosophers.[4] However, the quote from Horace
above suggests that the core concept of American bioethics that of individual
autonomy, is at least two thousand years old in Western thought.

Howard Brody, a leading American bioethicist, notes that bioethics
gained credence through two factors: the rising moral dilemmas of modern
technology and the problem of physician paternalism.[5] So far in this book I
have discussed several conundrums of medical technology. Vestiges of physician paternalism still persist when doctors present treatment options in a
manner that is biased toward their own repertoire of reimbursable interventions. Despite that, there is general agreement in bioethics and healthcare law
that paternalism is morally wrong, and the patient has the ultimate right to
decide what is or is not done to her/his body.[6]

Brody goes on to note that the clinical bioethics consultant, by expressing
the view that the patient's opinion must take priority, might elicit a negative

response from the physician planning a diagnostic or therapeutic intervention. Observing that medical practice tends toward a positivist and reductionist approach, he captures the dilemma of the bioethicist caught in the middle, accused by the medical specialist of limiting his/her intervention on one hand, and by critics of bioethics claiming that they legitimize the medical-industrial complex on the other.[7] Liberal deontological perspectives have predominated in bioethics, emphasizing the rights of individual patients following a Rawlserian notion of liberty and the precedence of individual rights.[8] However, this approach has given free rein to the market economy of medicine. One could view this as a natural development in a postmodern consumerist society where the importance of community and societal concerns has largely vaporized, consumed in the flame of consumerist individualism.[9] Lyotard notes that capitalism as a matter of course in serving expanding commercial markets, encourages disintegration of the modern social bond.[10] Where has bioethics stood on this development? It has adopted a market compatible approach distancing of social bonds in favor of individual autonomy and so has given tacit approval to the minimalist ethos of consumerism. This has permitted bioethics to persist, even flourish for a while, and hold on in the challenging environment of a dominant consumerist business ethos.

AUTONOMY *SANS* RESPONSIBILITY

While there is not a single bioethics position it is fair to say that the communitarian perspective is not a popular perspective in bioethics circles. In such a communitarian vein, my coauthor and I[11] suggested a decade ago that the privileges that health insurance confers, both public and private, ought to be linked to some extent to the responsibility to complete an advance directive. Such a policy would help reduce some of the social, moral, and clinical entropy that occurs when a patient loses decisional capacity without completing a document that can designate a surrogate decision-maker and provide some guidance to crucial medical care decisions. The response of most journal editors and reviewers was one of disdain for entertaining such pragmatic notion of individual accountability and responsibility. Advance directives (AD) have failed to achieve a substantial completion rate nationwide despite efforts to do so. The continued low completion rate of advance directives inhibits their utility, application and effectiveness. In our article we made the recommendation to link the completion of advance directives to the time when health insurance is initiated or renewed by amending the Patient Self Determination Act. This would relocate the time and locus of AD completion from the emotional turmoil of hospital admission and acute illness to a calmer time when family members and other advisors could be consulted and involved. Actuating an increased utilization rate may require non-coercive incentives as well as education. Amending the Patient Self Determination Act to require providing advance directive forms at the initiation of health-care insurance rather than at the time of hospital admission, in conjunction with educational and/or incentives, could be more effective than the current situation. In the original version of that manuscript, Eiser and Weiss suggested a mandate for all people with health insurance to complete an advance directive, but this was viewed as too coercive so we relented and revised our recommendation to provide some modest benefit to completing a directive such as a discount on a gym membership. Is it unreasonable to ask all insured people who possess decisional capacity to consider the possible life circumstances that might befall them suddenly and to act providentially to designate a surrogate decision-maker and provide explicit directions under what circumstances she/he would want "heroic" measures or not? But in a consumerist ethos, providential thinking is impermissible as it may be conceived as offensive to the consumer who now has the power to influence institutional outcomes through the completion of satisfaction surveys mandated by CMS. Thus the ethos of consumerism is very much in force for healthcare, and bioethicists have not shown a willingness to challenge it. It would not be politically correct to do so. Few desire to take on the dominant consumerist values, even if these values serious impair societal functioning.

Catharine MacKinnon[12] notes that if postmodern thinkers have a responsibility to effect positive change with regard to any one thing, they should reconsider some of their armchair criticism of social movements for the equality of women and other groups. I concur with MacKinnon that postmodern thinkers are predominantly critical and short on positive recommendations, including any linkage of rights and responsibilities. Postmodern thinkers, who are also predominantly male, are proficient at recognizing the current cultural mythology but are considerably less adept at suggesting a path out of our current societal morass and moral confusion. If one starts with the assumption that consumerism is the paramount social value in healthcare, then it is difficult to develop a thicker notion of interpersonal responsibility, interdependence, and something approaching cost effective health policy.

THE POSSIBILITY OF COMMUNICATIVE ACTION

Health policy in the United States is facing a crossroads, as a burgeoning technology-driven medical practice is consuming an increasing amount of the gross domestic product. In 2009, healthcare expenditures comprised 17.6 percent of the GDP[13] and 54.2 percent of federal government spending. The potential to align health benefits with healthy behavior needs serious exploration to encourage the development of a healthier population than currently exists. For example, there already are healthcare insurance plans that reduce co-pays based on the completion of health maintenance activities and healthy lifestyles.[14] The American Cancer Society, the American Diabetes Association, and the American Heart Association have issued a joint brief on the subject of financial incentives to encourage healthy behaviors.[15] Behavioral economics suggests that such an approach is more likely to work than our current *laissez faire* approach.

Simply expanding healthcare benefits is no longer a viable financial option given the exponential growth of healthcare technology, aging demographics, and the expanding scope of medical services. Can stakeholders with current received values arrive at a consensus on such a different tack? Can a consumerist-focused bioethics deal with such concerns effectively?

Perhaps a communicative ethic can improve on the prevailing model. The theory of communicative action advanced by Jurgen Habermas is grounded in the recurring patterns of ordinary language usage.[16] This ostensibly pragmatic solution to the problem of knowledge creates the possibility of a rationally based society where consensus was conceivable. Jonathan Moreno indicated that this rich philosophical model of group consensus is still challenged by the particular aspects of the group interaction.[17] Interpersonal aspects of the interactions may reduce the rational aspects of any deliberation. Once again the Foucauldian insight suggests that power relationships can undermine or destabilize a rationalized consensus and social structure such as the one that Habermas has carefully constructed. Correspondingly, in the real world of healthcare decision-making, there is currently a reluctance to formally confer decision-making authority on ethics committees because of the thinness of common agreement in this era. By whose authority and with what training would a deliberation be constituted outside of the standard formal judicial system? Several years ago Eiser and Seiden suggested a policy whereby a hospital ethics committee, inclusive of clergy, patient and family could reach consensus regarding dialysis withdrawal through a careful, respectful, culturally sensitive iterative deliberation.[18] While it is possible that such processes occur in some instances, but this extensive deliberation is exceptionally rare in today's litigious society.

Mediation in bioethics consultation attempts to reduce conflicts in healthcare decisions through use of a "neutral" mediator. Dubler notes that bioethics mediation helps lead to "principled resolution," grounded in a mixture of deontological and utilitarian principles.[19] This has had genuine, if modest, impact in lieu of a thicker implementation of communicative action in postmodern times. Such small steps may be all that one can expect in these troubled times of discordant values.

WHEN AUTONOMY HURTS HEALTH

For the past few decades there has been a forceful critique of the analytic approach to bioethics and principlism initiated by Danner Clouser and Bernard Gert.[20] The principles that were espoused and then applied analytically were patient autonomy, beneficence, non-malfeasance, and justice, with autonomy taking precedence over the others. Beauchamp and Childress, authors of the widely cited bioethics reference book,[21] interpreted autonomy as the individual's ability to plot their own course of action regarding diagnostic and treatment plans. Azetsop and Rennie, with a view of bioethics from Africa,[22] note that Kant's categorical imperative is not synonymous with bioethics' view of autonomy for Kant viewed moral agency as tied to a search for universalizable truth and respectable conduct. They further posited that American-Anglo bioethics comes closer to the views of John Stuart Mill, emphasizing the freedom of choice by the individual in a libertarian mode.

The patient autonomy by proxy by healthcare surrogates that prevails in the United States often leaves nurses and physicians, especially in intensive care units, feeling as though they are being treated as a means and not as conscious, sentient individuals violating in some fashion the categorical imperative. For example, nurses and to a lesser extent physicians have been cursed at and otherwise demeaned by disgruntled family members of patients who take exception to their clinical care or are simply angry about other aspects of their lives. Often mental illness, addiction, or family strife make the exercise of autonomy perilous to patient and provider alike. The excessive focus on autonomy thins out the moral content and the shared network of values between patient and provider.[23] Azetsop and Rennie also note that by emphasizing autonomy, bioethics has become consonant with a consumerist model and commodification of medical practice. While some bioethicists are explicit in embracing a libertarian, market-based perspective,[24] even the many who give emphasis to the liberal perspective are giving tacit approval to the market-driven commodification of healthcare. I observed nearly a decade and a half ago, "combining often unlimited commercial or government entitlements with unbridled autonomy produced a runaway consumption of healthcare."[25] At the time I had in mind a patient in our nephrology practice in New York City who continued for years to need emergent dialysis, hospitalizations for sepsis, and repeated vascular surgeries until he ran up a healthcare bill in the millions, often inconveniencing other patients as well as the professional staff. Patient autonomy assured him of the right to continually make poor personal choices regarding his health and demand emergent treatment, at some level, competing with the needs of other patients. Fifteen years later, a $2.7 trillion healthcare industry serving autonomous patients not incented to engage in health-promoting lifestyles or otherwise conserve their health is still an ethical conundrum that few, including bioethicists, want to confront.

Azetsop and Rennie also note that from the global perspective of a third world resource-poor country, autonomy-focused bioethics diminishes notions of public and community health, and renders social causes of illness invisible. Moreover, an autonomy-based ethic actually promotes the "perpetuation of the social status quo within which risks for poor health are greater."[26] Has a Western libertarian bioethics failed to account for a just distribution of clinical resources? Has it contributed to the social entropy of the clinical encounter as well as the added costs of care that may be futile? I believe it has.

SOCIOLOGY AND BIOETHICS CONFLICT: WHOSE PRINCIPLES AND WHOSE BIAS?

Several authors have observed a brewing antagonism between bioethics on the one hand and the sociology of medicine on the other. Hoeyer notes that sociologists of medicine feel their insights could inform bioethics regarding bioethics' own hegemonic views.[27] To support this view, Hoeyer cites Foucault's comment that the object of choice in a decision is never entirely voluntarily decided,[28] but is based on prior conditions and is contingent on various power relationships. Complete freedom of choice is quite ephemeral. Hoeyer also observes that sociologists have to some degree unfairly categorized bioethics as a homogenized monolithic entity when it is hardly so. He concludes that a dialogue between the two disciplines could be enriching to both, and I concur wholeheartedly while recognizing the difficulty of getting consensus from such a dialogue with both sides having vested interests and staunch positions.

Turner calls attention to the "debunking style" of the social scientist, disabusing bioethicists of their "specialness."[29] Bosk unmasks altruism as self-interest disguised,[30] while DeVries asks bioethicists to reflect how much they have compromised their own values in order to work in the biomedical industrial complex.[31] Interestingly, Bosk's observation regarding altruism is supported by neuroscience research indicating that altruistic and cooperative human acts are associated with activity in the brain's pleasure or reward centers.[32] When a person believes that she has conducted herself morally, she experiences pleasure via activation of a pleasure center in the brain. This does not equate moral conduct with other pleasurable experiences, but rather points out that other delineating principles are needed to define an act as moral. The moral thinness of consumerist culture renders such delineating principles elusive.

Turner challenges such sociological critiques, noting that bioethicists are quite a diverse group of thinkers with some quite critical of the biomedical industries. He further observes that sociologists have their own form of principlism or received wisdom, and finally notes that bioethics has expanded well beyond the focus on the patient-physician relationship. In other words then he posits that the reductionist view of bioethics held by some sociologists is a "straw man" critique, and I perceive the validity of his claim.

Brody gives consideration to whether bioethics can be engaged and activist.[33] He notes the insights of Judy Andre and Lisa Parker that bioethicists can and should have an activist voice in reducing power inequalities. Brody appears to suggest a middle way: that of cautious, reflective activism, lest bioethicists act prematurely before due deliberation. These arguments for greater moral activism also resonate to the sociologist critique of bioethics. But it is reasonable to ask how prophetic a voice can any profession in America maintain and still survive economically. Bauman offers some insights into the problems facing the moral self in a postmodern lifeworld:

"the moral self is the most evident and prominent among technology's victims. The moral self cannot and does not survive fragmentation. . . . In the universe of technology, the moral self, with its negligence of rational calculation, disdain for practical uses, and indifference to practical uses and indifference to pleasure feels and is an unwelcome alien."[34]

Thus it will not be easy to chart a course for the deliberative activist in a postmodern consumerist technosociety with less tenure and academic freedom and more corporate influence in the university. Critique alone, with which postmodernism is well endowed, cannot restore solidarity, a critical prerequisite, in my estimation, to ethical conduct. Bioethics' challenges are real and culturally dependent, embedded in our postmodern technosociety. Our culture can be held accountable for lacking an ethical ethos or dwelling in a simulation of reality that ignores serious moral problems. Who is accountable for the content and quality of our culture, shared or disputed values, and adoration of computerized technology? While government, politicians, corporate leaders, marketing departments and news media all have *de facto* roles in forming the ethos, there is a need for more informed deliberative discussion of the *why's*, *how's* and *wherefore's* of the content of postmodern culture, including and especially our medical culture. Perhaps Steve Jobs is not the best role model in America, visionary postmodern marketer that he was. Who will lead the post-postmodern movement?

Turner has noted that bioethicists have been oblivious to their own received philosophical assumptions, failing to note their own particularistic views, so that their pronouncements are much less generalizable than they are inclined to assume.[35] The reality of multiple interpretive communities seems to get glossed over in the principilist approach. But casuistry also requires shared narratives and tacit knowledge in order to reach some type of consensus, even as it is case-based. So the postmodern critiques of lack of overarching shared narratives, and the pluralistic nature of culture in an era of globalization still needs to be fully digested and addressed in the realm of bioethics.

Dan Callahan, co-founder of the Hastings Center for Bioethics, observed that the conundrum concerning the pluralisms of epistemes that exist in bioethics today create the particularism versus universal principle dilemma.[36] He views it as a standoff with neither aspect gaining the upper hand. He notes that, "all cultures deserve our presumptive respect, but none can claim a moral exemption from scrutiny and evaluation."[37] The same can be said of philosophical traditions including postmodernism as well as principlism and pragmatic bioethics. None of these philosophies should have a "free pass" without the proper scrutiny of some type of validity if applied to societal ills.

Are we left with a relativist quicksand of differing pluralistic traditions that cannot communicate with one another on a meaningful level? Moreno suggests one possibility is consensus whereby agreement is achieved by transforming the understanding of differing members of a communicating group.[38] However, there is no guarantee that all parties will agree to a common methodology and moral language. Durante suggests another solution by invoking a combination of the concept of episteme as the cultural-historic context of a truth claim, and Stout's insight that different epistemes from different traditions may nevertheless reach similar conclusions especially when abetted by Stainaker's[39] notion of "bridging concepts" that help create a guide or framework for reaching similar conclusions from different epistemic or religious tradition origins. The thinkers develop frames of reference that guide them in seeking common ground among divergent traditions. The process is discursive and iterative bringing to mind the work of Charles Pierce a century earlier whereby a community of interpreters of data and symbols recursively interprets its meanings.[40] Of course such a process requires patience and equanimity which is can be difficult to achieve in our frenetic "liquid postmodern" world. The superficiality of *hyperreality* that has become characteristic of contemporary life works against developing a moral consensus or sensibility of any thickness. The result includes a lack of civility that is growing in the medical world as well as other social realms in America as well as in other countries. Can these trends be countered effectively?

COMMUNITARIAN BIOETHICS AND POSTMODERNISM

Dan Callahan noted a decade ago that bioethics tended toward liberal individualism and needed a competitive voice that spoke to the common good, communitarianism.[41] He held that communitarian thought could reinterpret the four principles of bioethics with an eye toward a broader and thicker view of the good in autonomy, beneficence, nonmalfeasance and justice. Ironically, in the 2000 election, I recall both Bush and Gore paying "lip service" to communitarianism as both parties saw something of value in it, although no doubt differently.

I participated in the Communitarian Summit in February 1999 organized by Amitai Etzioni and others and spoke at the conference on a vision of the communitarian Health Maintenance Organization (HMO) where the community of patients participated in the policy decisions of the insurance company. As a prediction, my rumination was decidedly off the mark. However in the early 1980s participatory deliberative health plans existed in Group Health of Puget Sound, a smaller HMO in Evanston, Illinois, and others elsewhere. What happened to these instances of communitarian health policy? The forces of radical individualism, the demands of corporate capitalization, the juggernaut of technological advancement, and the indifference of postmodern society where entertainment and amusement (aesthetics) have trumped civic engagement that required time, deliberation, and effort. Civil society requires a degree of participation and responsibility that seems anathema to postmodern consciousness of leisure hedonistic pursuits, satire, and narrow particularism. More recently, Etzioni described a responsive communitarian bioethics that seeks to balance common good with autonomy through informal social controls, persuasion and education.[42] While that is a worthy consideration, it is difficult to actualize in our postmodern, individualistic, consumerist world. Today it is nearly impossible to find a strong voice for "society" in any sphere of social life; this is especially true in healthcare, where there are many diverse interest groups often not engaged in a mutually respectful dialogue. Online blogs and websites that are commonly used today actually discourage the face to face encounter that Levinas and Bauman have indicated is so important to the development of a personal sense of responsibility. In cyberspace we may feel connected but not so responsible for one another. Certainly pockets of communitarianism persist throughout the world, including in the United States, and will continue to do so. However the postmodern fluid ethos has prevented it from becoming a rising model for public policy. Moreover, American bioethics has enshrined autonomy so firmly in a power position that communtarianism has not developed into a substantial counterforce. The titles of two notable books on historical and bioethical aspects of healthcare, *Strangers at the Bedside*[43] and *The Care of Strangers*,[44] denote the current state of *anomie* in the clinical encounter where providers and patients do not identify themselves as part of the same communities. Royce, as well as Pierce, over a century ago identified that a community must share an interpretation of symbols, events, and meanings to experience being part of a community.[45] Patients, physicians, healthcare executives, patients, nurses, and bioethicists all use different symbols and interpretations regarding illness and healthcare. Thus if a communitarian approach were viewed as desirable, the prerequisites to its existence would have to be developed because they are missing in the twenty-first-century ethos. Can we learn and adopt a common language of values in healthcare? Possibly so, but this would require an organized effort to expand the communication among all the stakeholders and redistribute the power equilibrium.

POSTMODERN VIEW OF EMPIRICAL BIOETHICS

Ashcroft offers a postmodern "archaeology of bioethical knowledge" in the mold of Foucault and Lyotard.[46] He describes a first phase involving the discovery of bioethical problems and self-reflection on them, a second phase where philosophic analysis is applied to the problems, and a third phase where empirical research in ethics is performed using the methods of sociology. He suggests, in a manner reflecting Lyotard, that bioethics is engaging in a language game to find the proper use of empirical information with bioethical meaning. He goes on to indicate, in a fashion after Foucault that power relationships implicitly enter into the interpretation of the data. Noting that there is an implicit political component to the interpretation of survey results Aschroft states, "Empirical bioethics can perhaps best be understood as a sort of politics. . . ."[47] Having participated in such research including using the innovative methodology known as Q-sort,[48] I found this statistical technique permits one to minimize some of the subjectivity of interpretation but certainly not to eliminate it. Our study included the factor analysis of physician end-of-life decision-making; it began with seventeen different viewpoints and through analysis narrowed it down to three perspectives: patient-focused beneficence; patient and surrogate-focused beneficence, and substituted best interest of the patient. Since correlations in such sociological research rarely approach unity, subjectivity is essential to the interpretation. (Incidentally we also found in this study that physicians used a method of bioethical decision-making closer to casuistry than principlism.) Perhaps it is better to acknowledge this central insight of postmodern thought that social data is always subject to interpretation, language games, and power dynamics, and that a bias of one's own approach to the interpretation of data and symbols always persists to some degree. By making the implicit, subjective interpretation explicit, one can possibly advance human understanding; at the same time, it is also important to recognize its limits. Hopefully such honesty will prove beneficial in the long run for a more accurate understanding of empirical bioethics research, and perhaps for both bioethics and healthcare policy as well.

THE PROBLEM OF CULTURAL AND ETHICAL RELATIVISM

Brody notes the difficulty of constructing a universal principlistic approach to bioethics in a culturally and ethically pluralistic world.[49] He indicates that there are some common intuitions of fairness that even the moral relativist resorts to when pressed. He makes passing reference to the neo-pragmatist Richard Rorty. Rorty, while ceding the ineluctable contingency of truth, advocates for what is tantamount to a "leap of faith" to embrace "human solidarity" in order to maintain his liberal intuitions.[50] Morality then assuredly has both intuitive (emotional) and cognitive elements, and one must recognize and respect the distinction as Levinas did.

In the chapter on Violence and Transcultural Values in the book *Violence Against Women: Philosophical Perspectives*, I wrote that the desire for healthiness could be considered a universal principle at least when people are experiencing symptomatic illness.[51] This is probably true on the emotional level if not the cognitive one. Drawing on my experience as a nephrologist serving in New York City's most multi-cultural neighborhoods, I noted that people from diverse cultures repeatedly sought out Western allopathic medicine "despite its rigors, because of a tacit agreement in its efficacy. Although this approval is not without ambivalence, it is nevertheless meaningful." There are many ways of being sick and many types of cures but the consistent turning to Western allopathic medicine when seriously ill speaks of some type of universal desire for wellbeing and an endorsement of empirically-based medical practice. Very few patients were willing to rely solely on older ritualistic healing practices.

Harris,[52] seeking a scientific basis for morality finds that which maximizes human wellbeing and flourishing as defining that which is moral. He also seeks to amend the age old injunction against basing moral statements on scientific ones. While such an approach remains debatable, it is certainly worthwhile investigating. James Q. Wilson[53] noted that there are cultural universals, such as the social concept of social reciprocity and fairness, that are essential to all cultures because this type of cooperation is needed for human survival. Brown posits several universals with human reciprocity a principal one.[54] Thus it may not be that farfetched to develop a science of morality even if it strikes the ethicist as misguided. Harris suggests the structure of the brain may hold some answers as the neural structure of social cooperation has been described.[55] Clearly, moral relativism is a concern from the perspective of social cohesion, so an empirical study of morality may offer a positive antidote to moral confusion in postmodern technosociety. Jagodzinski noted while speaking of pedagogical ethics that Buddhism evokes an ethics through meditative self-examination of personal addictive desires that can then lead to increasing sensitivity to the Other.[56] Perhaps meditative self-examination can accomplish some of things needed that philosophy and bioethics alone cannot do. Human survival and flourishing will require some creative solutions that can achieve some type of simulation of moral consensus if it cannot be achieved through more traditional discursive processes. Perhaps the insights of Buddhism, that are primarily psychological in nature, can supplement a science of morality. I hold some hope that an interdisciplinary approach encompassing bioethics, sociology, evolutionary psychology, other types of psychology, and neurosciences can yield an amalgam that advances societal understanding of the problems of ethical decision-making including those in the biomedical realm.

SUMMARY

The power equation of modern bioethics, both liberal and libertarian in its perspective, has given autonomy a place of primacy above beneficence while having diminished the authority of the physician. Sociology has challenged bioethics to provide the most insightful critique of medicine citing both bioethics own tacit assumptions and its coziness with power elites. The principilist versus casuist debates have elucidated matters to a limited extent. As a counterweight to radical individualism and libertarianism, communitarian bioethics has made an effort but the weight of postmodern culture with corporate authority, technological advancement, and consumerist focus have substantially limited such an approach. The cultural and moral relativism of the postmodern world are challenging to developing an ethos of caring in healthcare. Even so, a renewal of cultural values may be possible through a multidisciplinary empirical approach to challenging conventional wisdoms and finding a path to a limited consensus rooted in empirical, reflective, and discursive approaches and by stretching and strengthening the intuitive aspects of the moral imagination. Pragmatic reconstruction of a thicker notion of the moral good may benefit from a multi-disciplinary approach that nurtures a fuller notion of the common good while preserving individual human values. The need to develop a thicker notion of the common good is great for a rational approach to dealing with the crises of healthcare delivery in postmodern America. The Levinasian understanding of an intuitive awareness of responsibility for the Other may serve as an important model to strive toward in healthcare delivery. Advances in a variety of social sciences, humanistic studies, neuropsychology, and neuroethics may help us develop a new and improved understanding of moral reasoning and intuition in the twenty-first century. There are possibilities for a thicker dialogue and understanding of human caring and connectivity.

NOTES

1. Horatio Flavus Horace. Odes.

2. MacKinnon C. A., Points Against Postmodernism, *Chi.-Kent L. Rev 75:*687–88:2000.

3. Bauman Z. Postmodern Ethics Oxford: Blackwell, 1993, p. 84.

4. Jonsen A. R. *The Birth of Bioethics.* New York: Oxford UP, 1998.

5. Brody H. *The Future of Bioethics.* Oxford: Oxford Univ Press, 2009 p. 27.

6. Schneider C. *The Practice of Autonomy: Patients, Doctors, and Medical Decisions.* Oxford: Oxford University Press, 1998.

7. Brody, Ibid.

8. Daniels N., Sabin J. *Setting Limits Fairly: Can We Learn to Share Medical Resources?* New York: Oxford University Press, 2002.

9. Bellah R. N., Madsen R., Sullivan W. M., Swidler A., Tipton S. M. *Habits of the Heart: Individualism and Commitment in American Life.* Berkeley: Univ Calif. 1986.

10. Lyotard J.-F. *The Postmodern Explained*, trans. Julian Perfnanis, Morgan Thomas. Minneapolis: Univ Minnesota Press 1993, 72.

11. Eiser A. R., Weiss M. The Underachieving Advance Directive: Recommendations for Increasing Advance Directive Completion. *Am J Bioethics.* 2001 Fall 1(4):W10

12. Catherine MiKinnon, Ibid.

13. Martin A., Lassman D., Whittle L., et al. Recession contributes to slowest annual rate increase in health spending in five decades. *Health Affairs* 30(1):11–22, 2011.

14. Healthy Blue Living. http://www.mibcn.com/pdf/employer/HBLWhatAreYouPaying. pdf Accessed July 7, 2011.

15. Financial Incentives to Encourage Health Behaviors. http://pulse.ncpolicywatch.org/wp-content/uploads/2009/11/PolicyStatement-AHA-ACS-ADA2.pdf Accessed February 26, 2011.

16. Pusey M. *Habermas* London: Routledge, 1987.

17. Ibid. Pusey 104.

18. Eiser A. R., Seiden D. J. Discontinuing dialysis in persistent vegetative state: The role of autonomy, community, and professional agency. *Amer J Kidney Dis* 30:291–6, 1997.

19. Dubler N. N. A "Principled Resolution": The Fulcrum of Bioethics Mediation. *Law and Contemporary Problems.* 74:177–200, 2011.

20. Clouser K. D., Gert B. A critique of principlism. *Journal of Medicine and Philosophy* 15(2):219–236.

21. Beauchamp T. L., Childress J. F. *Principles of Bioethics.* New York: Oxford Univ Press 1979.

22. Azetsop J., Rennie S. Principlism, medical individualism, and health promotion in resource-poor countries: Can autonomy-based bioethics promote social justice and population health? *Ethics and Humanities* 5:1, 2010. http://www.peh-med.com/content/5/1/1 Accessed February 1, 2011.

23. McCormick R. Bioethics, a moral vacuum. *America* 180:21–25, 1999.

24. Engelhardt T. H., Jr. *The Foundations of Bioethics.* New York: Oxford U P. 1986.

25. Eiser A. R. Communitarian Bioethics: Reasons for Optimism. *Responsive Community* Spring 1997; http://www.gwu.edu/~ccps/rcq/issues/7-2.pdf. Accessed July 7, 2011.

26. Azetsop p. 7.

27. Hoeyer K. "Ethics Wars": Reflections on the Antagonism between Bioethicists and Social Science Observes of Biomedicine. *Human Studies* 29:203–227, 2006.

28. Foucault M. *The Order of Things: An Archeology of Human Sciences* New York: Vintage, 1994.

29. Turner L. Anthropological and Sociological Critiques of Bioethics. *Bioethical Inquiry.* 6:83–98, 2009.

30. Bosk C.L. Irony, ethnography, and informed consent. In *Bioethics in social context*, ed. Barry Hoffmaster 199–220. Philadelphia: Temple Univ. 2001.

31. DeVries R. How can we help? From "sociology in" to "sociology of Bioethics." *Journal of Law, Med, Ethics* 32:279–292, 2003.

32. Rillings J., Gutman D., Zeh T., Pagnoni G., Berns G., Killts C. A neural basis for social cooperation. *Neuron* 35(2):395–405, 2002.

33. Brody, Ibid. 223–225.

34. Bauman Z. *Postmodern Ethics*. Oxford: Blackwell, 1993, p. 198.

35. Turner. Ibid.

36. Callahan D. Universalism and particularism: Fighting to a Draw. *Hastings Center Report*. 30(1):37–44, 2000.

37. Ibid. 41.

38. Moreno J. *Deciding Together: Bioethics and Moral Consensus* New York: Oxford University Press. 1995, p. 45.

39. Stainaker A. Comparative religious ethics and the problem of 'human nature'. J Religious Ethics. 33(2):187–224, 2005.

40. Pierce, C.S. (1868), "Some Consequences of Four Incapacities," *Journal of Speculative Philosophy* 2 (1868), 140–157.

41. Callahan D. Individual Good and Common Good: a communitarian approach to bioethics. *Perspective in Biology and Medicine* 46(4):496–507, 2003.

42. Etzioni A. Authoritarian versus responsive communitarian bioethics. *J Med Ethics* 37:17–23, 2011.

43. Rothman D. J. *Strangers at the Bedside: A History of how law and medical ethics transformed medical decision-making* New York: *Basic Books*, 1991.

44. Rosenberg C. *The Care of Strangers: The Rise of America's Hospital System*. New York: Basic Books 1987.

45. Oppenheim Frank M. A Roycean response to the Challenge of Individualism. In *Beyond Individualism*. edit Donald L Gelpi. Notre Dame, IN: Univ Notre Dame Press, 1989, 87–112.

46. Ashcroft R. E. Constructing Empirical Bioethics: Foucaldian Reflections on the Empirical Turn in Bioethics. *Health Care Analysis* 11(1)3–12, 2003.

47. Ibid. p. 12.

48. Wong W., Eiser A. R., P. S. Heckerling, R. Mrtek. Factors Involved in Clinical Ethical Decision-Making: Results From A Study Using Q Sort Methodology. *American Journal of Bioethics* 4: W-W22, 2004.

49. Brody H. *The Future of Bioethics*. New York & Oxford: Oxford University Press, 2009. Cross Cultural Concerns, chapter 7.

50. Rorty R. *Contingency, Irony, and Solidarity*, New York: Cambridge Univ Press. Chapter 9. Solidarity.

51. Eiser A. R. "Transcultural aspects of violence" in *Violence Against Women: Philosophical Perspectives* edit. S. French, W. Teays Cornell University Press 1999.

52. Harris S. *The Moral Landscape: How Science Can Determine Human Values*. New York: Free Press, 2010.

53. Wilson J. Q. *The Moral Sense*. New York: The Free Press, 1993, p. 65.

54. Donald E. Brown. *Moral Universals*. New York: McGraw Hill, 1991, p. 108.

55. Rilling J. K., Gutman D. A., Zeh T. R., Pagnoni G., Berns G. S., Kitts C. D. A Neural Basis for Social Cooperation. *Neuron* 35:395–405, 2002.

56. Jagodzinksi J. The Ethics of the "Real" in Levinas, Lacan, and Buddhism: Pedagogical Implications. *Education Theory* 52(1): 81–96, 2002.

Chapter Eleven

Ethical Medicine, Performativity, and the Silicon Cage

"The collateral victim of the leap to the consumerist rendition of freedom is the Other as an object of ethical responsibility and moral concern." —Zygmunt Bauman [1]

"The principle that any object or any action is acceptable as long as they can enter into economic exchange is not totalitarian in a political sense. But in terms of language it is, since it calls for complete hegemony of the economic genre of discourse." —Jean Francois Lyotard [2]

PERFORMATIVITY AND THE SILICON CAGE

Medicine is becoming essentially a corporate systems enterprise in postmodern America, and the trend in that direction will likely accelerate as Accountable Care Organizations (ACOs) become the vehicle for new reimbursement models. ACOs are a form of healthcare financing that involves bundled payments to an integrated healthcare provider that places some of the risk of the cost of care on the provider side and includes some portion of payment dependent on scores in quality measurements. [3] It is the later component that helps distinguish ACOs from an earlier form of health insurance known as full risk capitation managed care. This new insurance vehicle has accelerated the need to form healthcare conglomerates and further diminishes the voice and role of the medical professional as healthcare delivery has become increasingly a highly capitalized corporate enterprise. The excessive cost of American healthcare is part of the national economic crisis and has provided the impetus to such a change in insurance methodology. Because the advances in medical technology are very expensive, as well as the need for aggregation of large quantities of capital, there is a need to shoulder financial risk in these new insurance vehicles.

The implementation of numerous computerized technologies including electronic health records and computerized order entry, digitized genomics and digitized monitoring[4] has advanced the corporate juggernaut and created what I call the Silicon Cage of healthcare. One can consider this as the twenty-first century successor to Max Weber's Iron Cage of bureaucracy from the early twentieth century. Weber's concept of the Iron Cage described the process whereby bureaucracy implements a sterile and stern rationality in the name of efficiency while reducing human agency and autonomy,[5] and thus invoking an element of "mechanized petrification."[6] The Silicon Cage emphasizes the digitized data-driven nature of medical bureaucracies and medical technology in the twenty-first century which is having a similar impact on the medical encounter that Weber described a century earlier in industry. Decisions that CMS has made regarding Medicare reimbursements for Electronic Health Records (EHR), Computerized Order Entry (CPOE), "Patient Centered" Medical Homes (PCMH), and Accountable Care Organizations (ACO) further enhance the corporate control of medical practice by requiring expensive computerization and bundling of payment and risk contracting by healthcare providers. In addition to bundling payments to providers, the ACO is a method of funding healthcare that will require collaboration among the many components of a healthcare system in a systematic and coordinated manner designed to improve quality of care while reducing costs. For many if not most clinicians, the private practice of medicine will be curtailed or disappear altogether, as physicians sell their practices to healthcare organizations or otherwise become subsidiary to them.[7] The question will remain in this world of large healthcare systems run by executives and bureaucrats, what will become of the moral character of medical practice and the nature of medical professionalism.

Consider for a moment another sphere of American life dominated by large heavily financed corporations, the Wall Street financial companies themselves. Former leaders of financial institutions, like John Bogle of the Vanguard Group, indicate their disgust with the improprieties now commonplace in the financial industry.[8] Lipman quotes another former Wall Street firm (Paine Webber) CEO, Donald Marron, as stating that the geometric growth of capital in the industry has seriously strained its business ethics.[9] Adam Smith's "Invisible Hand" of capitalism that restrains itself is now not only invisible but truly non-existent. The moral casuistry of a homogenous, rule-bound, communitarian society of England in Smith's era that he attributed to the Invisible Hand (of cultural values) is not in effect in the consumerist "liquid modern" postmodern society. The need for a moral societal framework for capitalism was lost on and by Milton Friedman[10] when he successfully promulgated the notion that ethics was unnecessary if the marketplace had free rein. This loss of moral tone in medical corporations is at least as likely to adversely impact medical corporations as it has done to financial ones.

Lyotard[11] cites Luhman that *performativity* of procedures and processes replaces the normativity of laws and ethical norms.[12] That has certainly occurred in the healthcare industry where billion dollar fines for Medicare fraud may be viewed as the cost of doing business for leading for-profit healthcare corporations.[13] Thus morality is viewed as obsolete in the performative world of the trillion dollar healthcare industry where return on investment prevails over all other values. The captains of the medical industry do not want to have physicians tell them how to run *their* business. Medical professionalism, as represented by professional medical societies does not have the clout to forcefully contend with the mega-corporations' influence over the fabric of clinical care policy, at least not in the lobbying halls of government or in the board room. Some physicians have joined the capitalist ethos willingly and run their practices as postmodern businesses wherein *performativity* dominates over *normativity*, and their medical businesses thrive in that model, especially for certain specialties like orthopedic surgery and radiology. The face of the Other, the caring component of healthcare delivery, is rarely noticed in such practices that focus on performativity as predicted by Lyotard. Yet other physicians and healthcare providers seek to bear the Hippocratic torch as refracted by the more contemporary insights of Levinas to honor their commitment to the Other. Physicians are a very heterogeneous group in postmodern times and probably always have been so. Sustained by a moral life force that defies the consumerist capitalism ethos, nodes of this "ethical antiquity" persist in isolated practices, while the majority fall someone between the two extremes.

The Silicon Cage places efficiency and performativity in a lofty status at the expense of professional autonomy and responsibility. For medical education performativity means training physicians as role players for medical institutions, analogous to Marshall's description, "fulfilling their roles at the pragmatic posts required by its institutions."[14] Performativity has a focus on shortened patient-physician contact often exacerbated by the physician interacting with the computer rather than the patient, increasing patient dissatisfaction and a distancing within the patient-physician relationship.[15] If you have experienced this as a patient or as a provider, you have felt the presence of the Silicon Cage.

SOME NOSTALGIC MEDICAL HISTORY

Is it fair to ask as medicine becomes increasingly a corporate practice with electronically digitized order sets and electronic health records, what is going to insulate and preserve its moral tenor and professional values? Consider the history of one HMO, Group Health of Puget Sound (GHPS). It began as a consumer-governed non-profit organization, a self-governing cooperative. This was met with resistance by the local county medical society which responded by barring GHPS physicians from joinng the society, other hospital staffs, and continuing medical education events.[16] Such resistance only gave way when the Washington State Supreme Court determined such acts were illegal restraint of trade. GHPS was one of the first medical groups to implement preventive measures like vaccinations against polio and pap smears to detect cervical cancer. It pioneered telephone call-in centers staffed by nurses and automated prescription refill services. As a cooperative, GHPS was governed by an eleven-person Board of Trustees of volunteer consumer members elected by their peers.[17] It continues to be a leader in innovation in healthcare delivery including the chronic care model and the PCMH.

Although governed by a board that featured consumer members, GHPS faced deficits when competing with for-profit network model HMOs that had lower fixed costs. Budget cuts in the 1990s were followed by implementation of electronic health records and patient centered medical home models in the early 2000s. Member trustees note that while a cooperative can be challenging to run, it has clearly championed clinical values that benefit patients not shareholders. It does provide an example of the benefit of reducing the profit motive from healthcare delivery for providing a good level of healthcare at a moderate cost.

Cooperatives of course require a communitarian perspective that is not readily found in many parts of the United States. For example, in the New York area all of the staff model HMOs disappeared by the end of the 1990s and it is difficult to imagine a cooperative thriving in that hyper-competitive, individualistic American city. Although some other cooperatives were started elsewhere, including Evanston, Illinois, most have disappeared long ago altogether or been absorbed by for-profit plans. The managed care expansion of the 1980s was the initial vehicle that cleared the field of the gentler version of health insurers, the cooperative insurers. It is highly unlikely in the current political and economic climate that there will be any reduction in the role of for-profit healthcare organizations, since they are firmly entrenched in the delivery systems as well as being powerful lobbying forces in the political realm. Instituting a national health insurance plan like the other Western countries may have been a desirable goal, but it seems totally unrealistic, given the reality of the political landscape in the United States in the twenty-first century.

The lack of moral consensus found in our political institutions may be rooted in brain structures and its development,[18] so we may be waiting a very long time for any type of reform along those lines. While I believe it would be beneficial to return health insurance to a non-profit status, it is hard to imagine a path to that change in the postmodern ethos of performativity and the vaporization of normativity.

HEALTHCARE CONSUMPTION AS A POSTMODERN CONCATENATION

The American bioethical ethos when it emerged in the 1970s and consolidated in the 1980s and 1990s was both libertarian (autonomous decision-making regardless its consequences for society) and socially liberal (encouraging robust government entitlements). This combination of values in conjunction with corporate and physicians' profit motives contributed to runaway consumption of healthcare. For example American are encouraged to eat gluttonously by the for-profit food conglomerates through a combination of clever application of food science and effective marketing,[19] while living sedentary lifestyles being entertained by digital entertainment media. At the same time, healthcare consumers expect and demand the complete correction of a wide variety of maladies by a flawless and caring healthcare system. The myth of the exalted physician is replaced by the myth of the flawless, digital healthcare delivery system, that penumbra of the Silicon Cage.

The bioethics movement and the accompanying healthcare legislation it helped to generate both recognized the declining moral agency of the physician and contributed to the decline in physician authority. This debunking of physician authority could be viewed as consistent with postmodern deconstruction. However, Foucault noted that the linkage between power and knowledge was an essential one, and posited that trying to separate the two is not possible. In addition debunking the myth of the physician has had its own untoward consequences. Phenomena such as physician burnout are rampant not only in the USA but in many other countries such as Japan, Germany, the United Kingdom and others as noted in chapter 9. Generation X and Generation Y (the Millenials) demand that their life have work/life balance but that is easier to state as an objective than to achieve in reality for medical professionals. It also takes a toll on the professionalism of medicine when one's familial duties are on an equal footing with professional demands. The increased patient handoffs among physicians are not only opportunities for error[20] but also devalue the face to face human exchange that formerly was a crucial part of the clinical encounter and the development of ethical caring for the patient. The patient-physician relationship that I and other physicians experienced in the 1970s and 1980s are difficult to establish for physicians coming of age in the postmodern era of deconstructed medical myths, flattened hierarchy, declining civility, and loss of mutual respect. I have noted earlier that electronic media desensitizes through its digital remoteness and Levinas' face-to-face encounter so crucial to a personal professional ethic recedes in such institutions as the Patient Centered Medical Home where the role of the physician is converted to team leader or perhaps merely team member. This may be good for team egalitarianism and the expression, at long last, of the unheralded talents of the clinical pharmacist, home care nurse, physical therapist, social worker, nutritionist, and others. Much of this would be a welcome change in and of itself. Eiser and Connaughton developed and published an experiential workshop for recently minted physicians to learn firsthand what exactly other healthcare providers have to offer patient care.[21] The full term consequences of a more interdisciplinary approach to medical practice is not yet known at this writing but a reduction in physician autonomy is likely to continue and effect the professional ethos. While American football did not suffer a decline when quarterbacks stopped calling the plays, football never made a claim to be a moral enterprise and does not provide a personal service. Medicine, at least to a considerable extent, did have such a claim and responsibility but so the question of the effect of the flattening hierarchy on the professional ethos remains a concern to be monitored.

One may ask have we replaced one myth, the physician myth, with another, that of the flawless, computerized corporate healthcare system? Once one adopts the systems theory approach and nomenclature, it becomes theoretically appealing to view systems as the paragon of efficacy, effectiveness, and performativity. It would be foolish to say that computerization will not yield some improvements, as it has in limited circumstances yielded some already. But the current body of evidence of the improvements is surprisingly modest at this stage.

Debunking physician mythologies may have been honest, important and necessary, and those are not going to be restored. In the next phase, one might ask how will the myth of the flawless computerized corporate healthcare system fare? Certainly there are several concerns[22] about the loss of confidentiality of medical records when they are digitized and available over the Internet as well as the social reconstruction of the clinical encounter by postmodern social influences. We need to admit we are on uncharted territory in the historical development of healthcare delivery.

Postmodern deconstruction of the physician myth reduces the patient-physician relationship to a mechanical, mercantile one devoid of the powerful healing of belief. The theurgic power of the clinical relationship that drew on divine forces has been drained from the clinical encounter because that power is heavily dependent on myth and its emotive power. The full consequences of this change are still unfolding. Castellani and Wear note that medical professional culture is comprised of the cumulative narratives that form the basis for social interactions.[23] I would add that it is crucial to the role-modeling that needs to occur during medical education and particularly during postgraduate medical education. Whether new myths can mature and our moral imaginations maintain some robustness in the current corporate bureaucratic milieu remains to be seen. Certainly a culture is more than its narratives but the moral and aesthetic values espoused in those narratives are crucial to the social fabric of society. Jameson notes the effacement of the boundaries between high culture and popular culture in postmodernism.[24] Does the popular culture in the twenty-first century support the notion of medical professionalism? Or has deconstruction of the physician myth, the flattening of hierarchy, the focus on work/life balance, and the exponential growth of online medical information rendered the physician-patient relationship deflated and foundering?

Some Potential Antidotes to the Silicon Cage

In a very un-postmodern positivist vein, I will now try to delineate some possible "antidotes" to the ethically restrictive ethos embodied by the Silicon Cage. It is important not merely to critique the present state of affairs but to point in the direction of some possible approaches to maintain the humanistic aspects of medical practice. While these suggestions have a positivist element, I offer them in the vein of a post-postmodern development.

COMPLEMENTARY AND INTEGRATIVE MEDICINE

Integrative medicine is the latest iteration of what was formerly known as alternative and complementary medicine in earlier forms and included a variety of techniques including herbal remedies, meditation, chiropractic, osteopathic manipulation, a variety of body techniques, acupuncture, Tai Chi, yoga, homeopathy, and Aruyvedic medicine. The phrase "integrative" denotes these approaches no longer should be considered mutually exclusive to allopathic technology-based medical practice. These techniques have varying degrees of effectiveness in various disorders but the Cochrane Collaboration on evidence-based medicine indicates effectiveness or probable effectiveness in several conditions.[25] These integrative techniques often invoke the theurgic effects that make the patient feel valued and uplifted compared to the cold uncomfortable imaging device or the invasiveness of endoscopic procedures or the aloof attitudes of some allopathic specialists. Often integrative medicine invokes a team approach. So the postmodern leveling of the medical hierarchy may enhance the prospects of integrative medicine. For example the old fashioned paradigm of the physician admonishing the patient to lose weight to reverse the metabolic syndrome may be done more effectively by a team consisting of a nutritionist, exercise physiologist, a naturopath, and a behavioral therapist.[26] One can envision an integrative patient home may be more effective and patient-centered than the currently implemented "patient centered medical home" that is strictly allopathic, heavily dependent on data downloads, rigid practice guidelines, and standardized but limited quality measures. This integrative home may improve the patient-provider relationship even if the allopathic physician is not directing all aspects of clinical care. An integrative medicine program at a Ford assembly plant significantly reduced narcotic prescription use while increasing meditation practice, with meditation possibly having other health benefits.[27]

These developments raise the possibility of offering patient-consumers a choice between a strictly allopathic medical home versus an integrative medical home. Perhaps choice can include more than an either/or option, with a spectrum of degrees of variation in such matters. The potential for "rhizomatic" organization structure, suggested by Deleuze and Guattari, raises the possibility of a more diverse structure to the patient centered medical home, rather than just one model that rigidly embraces the Silicon Cage of data entry, downloads, Pay for Performance, and other technically derived parameters.

PLAINTREE MODEL AND POSTMODERN AESTHETICS

The Plaintree Model of Healthcare was originated by a native of Argentina, Angelica Thierot, in reaction to the coldness she encountered in American hospitals.[28] The Plaintree Model attempts to humanize the inpatient hospital setting and make the patient an active participant in their healing and recovery.[29] As those authors posed the question, is this model of care "quality with a human face"? A retrospective evaluation suggests that it can improve patient satisfaction and length of stay, and reduce costs for patients receiving knee and hip replacements.[30] A qualitative study in Norway appears to lend some credence to the approach of improving hospital aesthetics primarily for its psychological benefit to the patient.[31] Yet another study suggests that such improved aesthetics can improve healthcare worker well-being and performance and enhance human interaction in the clinical encounter.[32] Clearly the postmodern emphasis on aesthetics and potential improvement in the well-being of patients and providers may well increase the interest in such an approach to healthcare. Even so, cost constraints will probably be a limiting factor.

MINDFUL MEDITATIVE MEDICAL PRACTICE

As noted in chapter 9, physicians in postmodern times are suffering a great deal of burnout including depersonalization or distancing form others. This harms clinician and patient alike. A thoughtful response to this has been developed by a group at the University of Rochester School of Medicine. They demonstrated that with an organized program that included an eight-week intensive period followed by a ten-month maintenance phase that included mindfulness meditation, self-awareness exercises, narratives of meaningful clinical encounters, appreciative interviewing, and didactic information with discussion. Their results included significant reductions in burnout and depersonalization, and improved empathy, resilience, mood and emotional stability.[33] This intervention was complex requiring the involvement of experienced facilitators, the commitment of the participating physicians, and grant funding.

Another study using a stress reduction program for hospital employees that included reducing institutional generated stress found significant (70 percent) reduction in malpractice claims in those hospitals that had implemented the program.[34] This implies that less stressed personnel can be more responsive to patient care matters.

Stress reduction and mindfulness medical practice in healthcare are ideas whose time may have come in the twenty-first century. Surely for them to grow will require local and national champions and a supportive administration, especially in the absence of grant support. These practices certainly share some qualities with integrative medicine but could be implemented in a manner compatible with allopathic practice. Stress reduction through meditation can be an important adjunct for patients to specific treatment for several medical disorders.

Mindfulness meditation can also benefit patients. Kabat-Zinn et al. found it helpful in reducing pain, improving mood, and reducing use of pain medication in patients with chronic pain.[35] Davidson and Kabat-Zinn et al.[36] demonstrated that mindfulness meditation could improve immune response to vaccine as well as activate parts of the brain associated with positive affect. Clearly postmodern science combined with the ancient technique of meditation and advanced technology can provide benefits for patients and providers alike, a rare win/win in today's environment.

SCHWARTZ CENTER ROUNDS: GROWING COMPASSION ONE CONFERENCE AT A TIME

Some physicians may not spontaneously respond to Levinas' call for responsibility to the Other. However an exciting method has been developed by the Kenneth B. Schwartz Center,[37] initially implemented at the Massachusetts General Hospital and now at over 300 hospitals and outpatient facilities around the nation. This approach involves conferences that focus on the non-clinical aspects of challenging cases so as to promote provider sensitivity to emotional aspects of medical care. As one who has been facilitating these conferences at a community hospital for the past several years, I can attest to their power. These conferences permit physicians, nurses, social workers, transporters, security guards, and other healthcare workers to share their most emotionally charged cases. The multi-disciplinary panelists present and comment from their differing personal and professional perspectives, and then respond to comments and questions from the audience who are supportive and collegial in their manner of questioning. The staff in the audience is encouraged to describe similar encounters from their experience and, if familiar with the case, to share their own emotional reaction to the challenging circumstances. A recently published analysis[38] of the impact of the Schwartz Center Rounds (SCR) indicates that in both retrospective and prospective studies, attending the SCR decreased perceived stress, improved the ability to deal with the psychosocial demands of care, and fostered greater teamwork. The participating staff noted an improvement in the organizational culture as well as greater focus on patient-centered care. The spirit of the healthcare providers appears more upbeat after they have shared their greatest personal professional challenges and communicated across disciplines.

I surmise that Levinas would very much approve of SCR. Face to face encounters with other caregivers can grow one's understanding and compassion for both challenging patients and each other. One can consider SCR as a means to enhance awareness of the face of the Other.

MEDICAL SCHOOL PREREQUISITES SHOULD INCLUDE ETHICS AND/OR BIOETHICS

The Liaison Committee on Medical Education (LCME) which accredits American and Canadian allopathic medical schools requires medical schools to teach "medical ethics and human values."[39] As a result all medical schools do provide some instruction in medical ethics for their medical students. Naturally this topic competes with many other subjects that are of a scientific and technological nature. I would recommend that medical students should be required to take a course in ethics or bioethics in their pre-medical studies as well. Some have suggested that college is not a good place to learn bioethics because it lacks a clinical orientation[40] and that is probably so in many colleges. But all undergraduate schools can offer a course in ethics and that should be a prerequisite to studying medical ethics in medical school. One should be conversant in the vocabulary of ethical discourse and ethical analysis and argument before approaching the specifics of medical ethics. Moreover students take their prerequisites seriously. Harvard Medical School implemented a new set of prerequisites while it requires biology, chemistry, mathematics, expository writing, and physics, it only recommends humanities and social sciences.[41] Johns Hopkins Medical School's new requirement adds twenty-four semester hours of humanities and social sciences and that is closer to what I am suggesting here although I am specifically referring to ethics study.

Notably the American Association of Medical Colleges (AAMC) under the leadership of Darryl Karch has recently announced that the MCAT examinations used for medical school admission will add components in the social sciences and critical thinking.[42] I applaud this modification and suggest making ethics as well as psychology required topics of study so that medical students know it is important to becoming a capable physician. Postmodernism denotes the importance of discourse, deconstruction, and semiotics. How better to be an ethical postmodern clinician than to be conversant in the discourse of ethical theories and the significance of symbols? Perhaps it won't make one moral or empathetic but it will give some currency to ethical concerns and at least a greater cognitive awareness of ethical concerns.

FORMULA RELATING PERFORMATIVITY AND HUMANENESS IN MEDICAL CARE

Consider the following formula as a heuristic device:

$$K = P \times H$$

P = Performativity in Medicine = Computerized Medical Data, EHR, CPOE, Checklists, Order Sets, Pay for Performance, Robotics

H = Humaneness = individualized caring, compassion for patients by healthcare providers, narratives of clinical caring and excellence, acknowledging the face of the Other, theurgic elements

K = numerical constant = related to the reciprocal nature of performativity with humaneness and normativity

In the above formula, I am posing the hypothesis that the formula $K = P \times H$ is essentially true, i.e., that as electronic performativity increases, there is a reciprocal decline in the humanness of medical practice. It may not be true and I cannot verify that it is the case. I would even go so far as to say I hope it is not entirely true. But I think it is a useful heuristic to pose the question as a concern. Increased performativity holds the promise of improving healthcare's precision and accuracy. Operative checklists have been shown to reduce adverse events in the operating room[43] and are an important example of useful performativity. Yet it is possible that as technological advances continue to accelerate, the Silicon Cage in a manner analogous to the Faraday Cage, keeps the "electrifying" humanistic element out of the clinical encounter. I often hear patients complain that in consulting a physician today, the physician seems more focused on inputting or obtaining data from the computer than engaging them in a face to face encounter. That is certainly not universally true; some surveys suggest patients are satisfied with their physicians' use of computers.[44] However, the art of medical history taking may be diminished by the electronic checklist approach. Medical history taking at its best is an interactive art. Computerized history taking, especially when it is designed to fulfill bureaucratic purposes, may lose details important to diagnosis. Once again the texture and fabric of medical care is varied and complex, so the approach of a checklist which may work well in the OR may not be as useful as obtaining a medical history which may require an informed free text approach. The science of medicine provides probabilistic knowledge of complex human illness but the physician who acts as healer must interpret it both clinically and emotionally for the individual patient.[45] Thoracic surgeon Dr. Carolyn Reed notes that American society places a remarkable premium on technology but in reality technology can sometimes be a hindrance in delivering the appropriate medical care.[46] I have noticed instances where too narrow a focus on imaging technology has distracted physicians from the patient's most pressing medical needs.

SUMMARY

Postmodern medical practice favors performativity over normativity, productivity over professionalism. The Silicon Cage comprised of electronic medical records, computerized order entry, and large healthcare bureaucracies are designed to maximize data collection and electronic surveillance of medical performance with an intention to reduce medical errors and maximize corporate profits. Does the enhanced performativity of twenty-first century medical practice diminish the humaneness of medical practice?

In a positivist vein, I have suggested some post-postmodern "antidotes" to the Silicon Cage: integrative medical practices that to some extent recapture the theurgic sense of healing; the Plaintree model that emphasizes both patient empowerment and improved aesthetics; mindful medical practice that incorporates meditation, self-reflection, and appreciative inquiry to reduce physician burnout and improve empathy; Schwartz Center Rounds to give currency to empathy and provide mutual support across the medical disciplines and professions. The AAMC mandates that future physicians be educated in medical ethics, and is now adding requirements for training in the social sciences and critical reasoning. The ethical practice of medicine is possible in the twenty-first century but it will require a great deal of innovative measures to enhance the humanistic practice of medicine. While Levinas can provide some postmodern guidance, a variety of approaches will be needed to influence a diverse physician and patient population. Cooperative non-profit health maintenance organizations with patient representation on the board of directors could help in generating a variety of formats for the patient centered medical home, from the fully digital and data-driven to the more integrative approaches. I suggest that there could a variety of types of medical homes with varying degrees of performativity and humaneness. I also suggest there may be an inverse relationship between the two, and raise the possibility of a post-postmodern ethos.

NOTES

1. Bauman Z. *Does Ethics Have A Chance?* Harvard U Press. P53.

2. Lyotard J-F. *The Post Modern Explained.* Transl J. Petanis, Morgan Thomas. Univ Minnesota Press, 1997.

3. Fisher E., et al. Fostering Accountable Health Care: Moving Forward in Medicare. *Health Affairs.* 28(2): 2009. 219–231.

4. Topol E. The Creative Destruction of Medicine: How the Digital Revolution will Create Better Healthcare. *New York Basic.* 2012.

5. Weber M. *The Protestant Ethic and the Spirit of Capitalism.* T. Parsons (trans.), A. Giddens (intro), London: Routledge, 1904–05/1992.

6. Kim S. H. Max Weber. *The Stanford Encyclopedia of Philosophy*, (Fall 2012 Edition), Edward N. Zalta (ed.). http://plato.stanford.edu/archives/fall2012/entries/weber/.

7. Harrison J. D. Healthcare law Driving Doctors away from small practices toward hospital employment. http://articles.washingtonpost.com/2012-07-19/business/35489044_1_primary-care-physicians-health-care-reform-law-accountable-care-organizations. Accessed May 15, 2013.

8. Lipman J. Are Ethics for Suckers? *C-Suite Newsweek* April 18, 2011. P 8.

9. Ibid p 8.

10. Friedman M. The Social Responsibility of Business is too Increase Profits. New York Times Sept 13, 1970.

11. Lyotard J.-F. *The Postmodern Condition: A Report on Knowledge.* Univ Minnesota Press, p. 46.

12. Luhman N. *Legitimation durchVerfahren.* Neuweid: Luchterland, 1969.

13. http://www.uow.edu.au/~/bmartin/dissent/documents/health/entry_to_Tenet.html accessed May 4, 2011; http://en.wikipedia.org/wiki/Hospital_Corporation_of_America

14. Marshall J. D. Performativity: Lyotard and Foucault Through Searle and Austin. *Studies in Philosophy and Education* 18:309–317, 1999.

15. Brownlee S. The Doctor Will See You—If You are Quick. *Newsweek* 46, April 23–30, 2012.

16. Kuttner R. Must Good HMOs Go Bad? The Commercialization of Prepaid Group Health Care. *NEJM* 338(21):1558–1563, 1998.

17. Tretheway B. E. A Brief History of Healthcare Cooperatives and Consumer-Governed Healthcare http://www.cooperativenetwork.coop/wm/coopcare/web/CLE%20-%20What%20makes%20a%20health%20care%20cooperative%20unique%20-%20MSBA%202011-04-15.pdf

18. Kanai R., Felden, Firth C., Rees G. Political orientations are correlated with brain structure in young adults. *Current Biology* 21: 1-4, 2011. DOI: 10.1916/j.cub.2011.03.017.

19. Kessler D. *The End of Overeating.* New York: Rodale, 2010.

20. Sen S., Kranzler H. R., Didwania A. K., et al. Effects of the 2011 Duty Hour Reforms on Interns and Their Patients. *JAMA Int Med.* Published online March 25, 2013. http://archinte.jamanetwork.com/article.aspx?articleid=1672284 Accessed May 16, 2013.

21. Eiser A. R., Connaughton J. Experiential learning of systems-based practice: a hands-on experience for first-year medical residents. *Acad Med* 83(10): 919–923, 2008.

22. Allen A. L. Confidentiality of Health Care Records. *Penn Guide to Bioethics* Spring 2008.

23. Castellani B., Wear D. Physician Views on Practicing Professionalism in the Corporate Age. *Qual Health Res* 10:490–506, 2000.

24. Jameson F. *Postmodernism and Consumer Society.* Verso: 1991, p. 193.

25. Cochrane Collaboratives: Complementary and Alternative Medicine; http://www.compmed.umm.edu/cochrane_about.asp.

26. Maizes V., Rakel D., Niemiec C. Integrative Medicine and Patient-Centered Care. *Explore* 5(5):277–289, 2009.

27. Kimbrough E., Lao L., Berman B., Pelletier K. R., Talamonti W. J. An Integrative Medicine Intervention in a Ford Motor Company Assembly Plant. *J Occup Environ Med* 52(3): 256–7, 2010.

28. Newsline for Pharmacists. http://www.news-line.com/featureone.lasso?-Search=Action&-token.profession=PH&-token.target=featureone&-Table=webinfo&-MaxRecords=50&-SkipRecords=0&-Database=press*&-KeyValue=223. Accessed May 16, 2013.

29. Blank A. E., Horowitz S., Matza D. Quality with a human face? The Samuels Planetree model hospital unit. *Jt Comm J Qual Improv.* 1995 Jun; 21(6):289–99.

30. Stone S. A retrospective evaluation of the impact of the planetree patient-centered model of care on inpatient quality outcomes. *Healthcare Envirom Res Design* 1(4): 55–69, 2008.

31. Caspari S., Eriksson K., Naden D. The importance of aesthetic surroundings: a study interviewing expert within different aesthetic fields. *Scandinavian J Caring Sciences* 25:134–142, 2011.

32. Rechel B., Buchan J., McKee M. The impact of health facilities on the healthcare worker's well being and performance. *Nursing Studies* 46(7):1025–1034, 2009.

33. Krasner M. S., Epstein R. M., Beckman H., Suchman A. L., Chapman B., Mooney C. J., Quill T. E. Association of an Education Program in Mindful Communication with Burnout, Empathy, and Attitudes Among Primary Care Physicians. *JAMA* 302(12): 1284–1293, 2009.

34. Jones J. W., Barge B. N., Steffy B. D., Fay L. M., Kunz L. A., Weubker K. I. Stress and medical malpractice: organizational risk assessment and intervention. *J Appl Psychol* 73(4): 727–1735, 1988.

35. Kabat-Zinn J., Lipworth L., Burney R. (1985). The clinical use of mindfulness meditation for the self-regulation of chronic pain. *Journal of Behavioral Medicine* 8(2): 163–190. http://en.wikipedia.org/wiki/Digital_object_identifier.

36. Davidson R. J., Kabat-Zinn J., Schumacher J., et al. Brain and immune activation produced by mindfulness meditation. *Psychosomatic Med* 65(4): 564–570, 2003.

37. Kenneth B. Schwartz K. B. Center for Compassionate Caregiving Website. http://www.theschwartzcenter.org/.

38. Lown B. A., Manning C. F. The Schwartz Center Rounds: Evaluation of an Interdisciplinary Approach to Enhancing Patient-Centered Communication, Teamwork, and Provider Support. *Acad Med* 85:1073–1081, 2010.

39. LCME Structure and Function of a Medical School E23 http://www.lcme.org/functions.pdf. Accessed May 2012.

40. Doukas D., McCullough L., Wear S. Reforming Medical Education in Ethics and Humanities by Finding Common Ground With Abraham Flexner. *Academic Medicine* 85(2):318–23, 2010.

41. http://hms.harvard.edu/admissions/default.asp?[age=requirements. Accessed May 15, 2011.

42. Karch D. https://www.aamc.org/newsroom/newsreleases/2011/182652/110331.html.

43. Haynes A. B., Weiser T. G., Berry W. R., et al. A Surgical Safety Checklist to Reduce Morbidity and Mortality in a Global Population. *N Engl J Med* 360(5):491–9, 2009.

44. Lefiever S., Schultz K. Does computer usage in patient-physician encounters affect patient satisfaction? *Can Fam Physician.* 2010 January; 56 (1) : e6–e12.

45. Lown B. *The Lost Art of Healing.* New York: Random House 119–120. 1999.

46. Reed C. E. Patient versus Customer, Technology versus Touch, Where has Humanism Gone? *Ann Thoracic Surg* 85:1511–1514, 2008.

Chapter Twelve

Medical Care Embedded in American Culture

Repositioning the Medical Ethos for the Twenty-First Century

"Rules would tell me what to do and when; rules would tell me where my duty starts and when it ends; rules allow me to say, at some point, that I may rest now as everything that had to be done has been done." —Zygmunt Bauman [1]

"Like it or not, the West has become a plurality of competing sub-cultures where no one ideology or episteme dominates for long. . ." —Jencks [2]

". . . medicine's finest hour is the dawn of its dilemmas. For centuries medicine was impotent. . . . Today with 'mission accomplished' its triumphs are dissolving in disorientation. Medicine has led to inflated expectations, which the public eagerly swallowed. Yet as those expectations become unlimited, they are unfulfillable: medicine will have to redefine its limits even as it extends its capacities." —Roy Porter [3]

LACK OF INFORMED PUBLIC ETHICAL DISCOURSE

There exists a deficit of ethical discourse in postmodern culture. Little public ethical discourse is ever seriously entertained in a philosophical manner; morality is strictly privatized, individualized, compartmentalized in personalized space, be it in the blogosphere or other such venues. The acrimony of political debate today reinforces the notion that there can be no dispassionate public discourse across the political spectrum. It is difficult to see how our society can address the difficult challenges of organizing medical care in this epoch without first improving the level of discourse of social values and ethical matters. This conceivably could be done by enhancing the education of all citizens with regard to philosophical concerns and methods in debating matters of great importance although education alone may not accomplish this goal. As McCollough notes,[4] in contemporary America, the emphasis is on efficiency, organization, technology, and profit leaves little room for serious moral deliberation on difficult subjects. The public sphere is subsumed by advertising, marketing, entertainment, partisan politics, electronic gossip, and other interests devoid of ethical orientation. Giroux has noted that schools in the twenty-first century have become venues for selling products instead of creating deliberative citizens.[5] We have ceded the *polis* to advertising in a variety of electronic formats.

How are we going to rationally discuss difficult healthcare issues concerning resource allocations, privacy of medical information, genomics, the impact of technology and cost effectiveness, if we do not learn the underlying philosophical and mathematical principles and the structural facts that impact these issues? There is a need to seek a higher level of public discourse and a greater understanding of the implications of ethical and statistical analysis in solving societal healthcare problems. Poses noted that large bureaucratic organizations, including the regulatory agencies, act in accordance with their own agendas and threaten to undermine the core values of medical practice,[6] as the physician turns into a technocrat controlled by various interlocking bureaucracies.

Postmodern thought has awakened us to the many changes in our social milieu over the past generation. Consumerism has created a very individualistic, legalistic, and commercial view of professional encounters in healthcare. The flattening of the medical hierarchy has vaporized the myth of the physician, leaving the physician vulnerable to criticism, sometimes founded and sometimes not. The exponential growth in medical knowledge requires both continuous learning and revision of standards that create anxiety and uncertainty as well as medical progress. The Foucauldian insight about the interaction between power and knowledge is clearly actualized in the realm of the medical-industrial complex.[7] As long as for-profit companies fund the research and advertise substantially in medical journals, detail their products to physicians, and pay honoraria and consulting fees, one shouldn't be surprised if the practice guidelines are skewed in the direction of more costly expenditures. Coupled with an atmosphere of fear of medical liability and fee for service profit alignment, performing more clinical interventions is often the case in postmodern American medical practice wherein patients often clamor for interventions after having seen advertisements them.[8] There is no sense of limits on societal resources, no sense of the need for a risk/benefit calculation. The ideology of radical individualism filled a void from the loss of communitarian moral standards and segues nicely with corporate capitalism and its consumerist ideology. The creation of the need for superfluous goods and services certainly extends to healthcare as well as more of the human condition becomes medicalized.

There is a need to change this paradigm through greater awareness of the judicious use of medical resources. This will challenge the medical consumerist ethos; comparative effectiveness research will only be a component of such an effort that requires more than merely more data analysis. Fact analysis alone will not resolve the issues of resource allocation because power/knowledge exigencies prevail. Just as consumerism has colonized pedagogy and the sphere of education,[9] so it has done to medical practice. Apropos to the excess of healthcare services, Baudrillard notes that consumer society is driven by excess capacity rather than genuine consumer need.[10] Postmodern analysis illuminates this healthcare dilemma.

Could raising the level of knowledge of ethical discourse starting with more ethics education in colleges and high schools help? Several authors contend that good public deliberation is possible but that structure and process must be developed and followed assiduously.[11] I do not think we have seen good examples of public deliberation regarding healthcare decisions since the Oregon Healthcare Decisions Act[12] over two decades ago. Postmodern culture may have made any such deliberations harder to attempt let alone accomplish.

Sternberg has both studied and advocated for the role of wisdom development in education.[13] His theories of wisdom education that balance self-interest with other-directed concern and tacit and formal knowledge were applied in a New Jersey school district with apparently very positive results for these students.[14] Why haven't such efforts become more widespread? The reason most likely relates to the fact that the pervasive consumerist ethos eschews contemplating the selfless, the deliberate, and the unexciting.

ALTRUISM AND ALTERITY

Attempts to retain the older concept of medical professionalism as grounded in a sense of altruism toward patients by physicians reflects a failure to denote the emerging estrangement that is increasingly common in the postmodern electronic clinical encounter. While older forms of altruism may still exist to some extent in some locales and practices, the prerequisites to the development of altruism are dissipating in the postmodern milieu. Studies indicate altruism is focused on those individuals who can be identified as part of an in-group.[15] Moreover we have learned that oxytocin release mediates much of altruistic behavior toward in-group members but not toward out-groups.[16] Thus the natural altruism of in-groups can no longer drive medical professionalism in the multi-cultural electronically dissociated twenty-first-century social milieu. Moreover, the flattening of the medical hierarchy reduces the robustness of altruism that previously arose from a sense of *noblesse oblige*.

Postmodern critiques of the myth of the physician further reduce the notion of medical practice as an extraordinary moral calling. Some postmodernist thinkers such as Levinas and Bauman counter relativism with a thick notion of responsibility to the Other. They note that this is an inherent human quality that transcends ethical theories and is intuitive and emotionally driven. Still they cannot deny that such a sense of responsibility for the Other is conditioned by the perception of similarity to self or in-group identity. Such sentiments can be diminished by electronic desensitization that is all too common today. The multicultural nature of American society, as well as global societies in general, will influence the strength of this sense of obligation to strangers at the bedside and in the clinic. Zygmunt Bauman noted that the *raison d'etre* of ethics is social cohesiveness and collaboration,[17] so it is truly vital for the well-being and preservation of a society to have a sense of moral value in its public sphere. The practice of medicine as well as medical education are dependent on the nurturing of an ethical ethos that is conducive to human cooperation in the clinical encounter as well as in other spheres of social life and discourse. The public sphere, and the ensuing consciousness that it evokes, has, however, been left to the consumerist capitalist marketing milieu. This has affected all spheres of postmodern social life including marriage, education, work life, and fashion as well as crime, drug abuse, distribution of wealth, and obesity. All the emphasis on consumerist autonomy leaves the individual without "protection from his desultory motivations."[18]

The growth of medical technology and the corporate control of medical practice create a further challenge to the practice of medicine as a holistic healing art. Rather these developments hold out a model of a purely rational, digitized vision of medical excellence that is heavily focused on clinical data, supervision, and control by internal and external bureaucracies. The assessment of quality, safety, computerization, and mechanization of processes have accelerated with both positive and negative impacts on the nature of medical practice. Despite rising healthcare costs, a mandate, both federal and private (Leapfrog Group), arose that computerization and mechanization must be better than the status quo and worth pursuing despite the substantial added costs and relatively little evidence of benefit. Serious deliberation on the cost of computerization of healthcare delivery has been deferred and is yet to be fully addressed.

If healthcare delivery continues to focus on digital data, it will continue to alienate patients and physicians who are seeking something more than mechanistic precision. Borgmann encourages us to consider the nature of technology interactions and not focus solely on the power of technology. He notes: "Technology . . . promises to bring the forces of nature and culture under control to liberate us from misery and toil . . . there is promise that this approach to reality will, by way of domination of nature, yield liberation and enrichment."[19] He further posits that this vision has led contemporary society to believe that technology is the key to the good life.[20] His insights help expose and understand the myth that unbridled medical technological growth is the answer to what ails healthcare. The CMS healthcare bureaucracy appears to subscribe to the dominant myth of the twenty-first-century viz., that more advanced technology inevitably leads to better outcomes as it implements "meaningful use of electronic medical records and orders."[21] The Leapfrog Group, a consortium of large employers, has taken a more cautious approach with concern that the EHR may be introducing new types of medical errors and views the matter with greater discernment.[22]

Levinas has provided an ethic for postmodern times: ethically commanded by the face of the Other whereby one experiences ethics prior to ontology prior to argument even prior to rationality.[23] He substantiates the experiential morality of sociability. He has inspired some bioethicists to reconsider bioethics in light of his philosophy. The existential difference of the Other, their alterity, cannot be overcome but remains an ethical call to those sensitive to this element. Such an ethical sensibility is hardly universal, especially in our multicultural world. Levinas held that science, technology and ontology cannot be prior to the moral sensibility. Clifton-Soderstrom notes that a Levinasian perspective has engendered the development of the birthing centers away from the interventionalist approach found in the traditional hospital setting where the human narrative gets subsumed in the name of technological advancement.[24] Technological intervention is nurtured by expectations of higher rates of successful outcomes but does not always deliver on this promise.

The maintenance of altruistic intuition and behavior requires gratitude in order to generate a sense of reciprocity.[25] Postmodern culture, however, is short on gratitude. So evoking the Face of the Other may be suppressed by the lack of reciprocal gratitude for deeds of an altruistic nature. Nurturance of optimal professional conduct needs a responsive patient, a more understanding bureaucracy, and a society with a thicker moral ethos. Patient surveys alone will not accomplish this but may be a partial component.

POSSIBLE POSTMODERN ALTERNATIVES TO AUTONOMY: CRITIQUE FROM AFRICA AND THE ICU

The focus on patient autonomy that has been at the heart of American bioethics for many decades developed as the communal moral standards evaporated in a sea of multiculturalism, individual rights, radical individualism, and the predominance of a consumerist model. Perhaps it takes a view from outside the United States to fully grasp what bioethical principlism and medical individualism have wrought. Azetsop and Rennie from South Africa observe that the promises of autonomy are unrealistic in any setting with limited resources. They view the conception of medical autonomy as a justification for market forces to dominate healthcare delivery.[26] They note "If we consider the patient as a potential victim *and* vector, we need to shift our gaze from the healthcare that might be most desirable for the individual patient to broader social concerns and the . . . distribution of care that might enable all to achieve opportunities over a reasonable life span."[27] This has been somewhat alien to the American perspective but even here questions are being asked about the limits of medical spending and the need to consider health from a population perspective.[28] Would "health-centered" medical care that puts patient health and rational understanding of a full life expectancy at the center make more sense than a consumerist model of medical care? Persad, Wertheimer, and Emanuel have put forth the "complete lives system" that involves prognosis as well as age and prioritizes the use of medical resource allocation to maximize the number of individuals living complete lives.[29] Is the current overconsumption of medical care a moral or social concern? For example, does performing chronic dialysis on and implanting automated defibrillators in nursing home patients fulfill appropriate goals of medicine? Do such patients ever give fully informed consent and would they do so if they could? These are very difficult but ultimately necessary questions.

It would also be necessary to articulate what constitutes a responsible patient and responsible surrogate decision-making. However, such constraints are antithetical to a consumerist autonomy model of healthcare delivery. The moral distress of intensive care nurses providing care in futile circumstances, when families of patients insist upon it, is substantial. Studies of ICU nurses revealed that half of them were experiencing moral distress from rendering intensive care that they regarded as futile and inappropriate[30,31] with many leaving working in an ICU or even the nursing profession.

Clearly, what is needed is a postmodern critique of the consumerist model. That critique would deconstruct, and examine the social and pragmatic implications of the autonomy principle rather than accepting it as received wisdom. Isn't it appropriate to consider developing a new model concerning medical decision-making near the end of life? Who is gazing on the face of the morally distressed ICU nurse or physician? Mannison and Hall, in their discussion of postmodern health economics, note that postmodern thought can raise important questions regarding "received canon" about power and exclusion as well as efficiency and equity.[32] Wilk notes that when affluence (or the affluence of insurance) isolates the individual from the consequences of their consumption, that moral controls on decision-making are lost.[33] Those morally distressing decisions in the ICU not only add to the patient's suffering when recovery is highly unlikely but also deprive someone else because there is no such thing as infinite economic resources in any society. Postmodernism inhibits the notion of a common good linking rights with responsibilities. I have suggested elsewhere that the right to healthcare and healthcare insurance should carry the responsibility to complete an advance directive.[34] Otherwise individuals may receive care that they themselves would not desire or benefit from simply because they did not prudently consider documenting their preferences in these serious matters.

Reflexivity calls attention to the interconnectedness of the observer and the observed, the healthcare provider and the patient. Foucault notes that each epoch has epistemes that are its collection of assumptions, implicit cultural values, approaches to problem solving, and so on.[35] We face the need to build new epistemes based on reflexivity (interconnection of observer and observed), collaboration, awareness of mutual need, potential for excessive amounts of healthcare spending, and the power and influence of the medical-industrial complex. Should a societal voice enter the dialogue? Politically it is daunting to see how such a voice of the common good can be located in the dissonance of competing political stances and special interests. Is a rigid, formulaic bureaucracy the only way to have a societal voice? Or can rhizomatic, self-organizing groups such as the "participative" HMO develop to fulfill this need? An enabling bureaucracy has features that include minimizing power asymmetries, procedures for balancing autonomy and responsibility, and flexibility with reliable application of rules.[36] It requires a style of leadership sensitive to the precariousness of this balance. I am not sure we have witnessed such balance yet in our regulatory or provider organizations. Nevertheless it may yet be possible to develop the sophisticated wisdom that is needed to truly advance the way healthcare is delivered in a humane, efficacious, and cost-effective manner.

If decision-makers are to avoid an egocentric approach, all must learn some ethical reflexivity so that one can recognize one's own received assumptions. Ethical reflexivity requires making ethical values and personal judgments explicit and most importantly weighing, as dispassionately as possible, the effects that one's values judgments may cause, including unintended harm.[37] All of this requires greater education in philosophy and the social sciences for those in decision-making status.

PATIENT ACTIVATION, ACCOUNTABILITY, AND THE NEED FOR REFLEXIVITY

Consistent with the postmodern notions of the flattened medical hierarchy, patient activation is a concept and a measurement technique that fosters and determines the degree to which patients are active participants in improving their health and treating their chronic conditions. Certainly in postmodern clinical encounters, many patients want to engage in their care in some meaningful fashion. More highly activated patients have knowledge of their illness, actively participate to improve their condition, and show a high degree of adherence to the medical regimen.[38] Supportive and continuous provider relationships with patients have been shown to correlate with measures of patient activation.[39] However, if the Silicon Cage model of processing and analyzing data at a great distance from the patient and the clinician continues to grow, then the encouraging development of patient activation may be thwarted. Borgmann has cautioned not to let technological knowledge run wild and overrun both culture and human nature.[40] What is the correct balance of analytic data and human interaction in medical practice? It is yet to be determined, but there is a need to seek such equilibrium.

Howard notes that Deleuze and Guattari warn against the homogenizing power of the new world order of domination as opposed to non-dominating rhizomatic relationships.[41] An example of such "rhizomatic" power in the medical realm is the recent patient-initiated observational study using the online social network Patients like Me to refute a published study that lithium carbonate is efficacious in amyotrophic lateral sclerosis (ALS). This is postmodern patient activation using social media technology in a novel and effective way[42] and suggests new possibilities in escaping from the bureaucratic Silicon Cage using social media. However, social networking can also spread misinformation and dissemble professional authority. This further flattening of the medical hierarchy may have both benefits and drawbacks; the new balancing of authority is yet to be worked out.

One could ask where is patient accountability in the development of the patient-centered healthcare model. Holding only physicians and nurses accountable and liable for outcomes and errors fails to recognize that patients share some responsibility for clinical outcomes with regard to regulation of diet, compliance with the medical regimen, and exercising restraint regarding risky behaviors. The face of the Other is difficult to visualize when reciprocity is lacking. On the other hand, shouldn't a collaborative and careful patient share in the recognition and reward for good outcomes including cost effectiveness? It is possible to devise a system that provides an alternative to a strict consumerist view of patients viewing them as responsible participants in their own healthcare. In fact, it is conceivable to view the current healthcare crisis of excess as resulting from that consumerist model. Detsky[43] observed that patients often have unrealistic expectations of healthcare services including the expectation of uniformly excellent outcomes, service with empathy, and little out of pocket expenses or lifestyle changes. While Detsky recommends that health policy needs to understand and respect consumer expectations, I am suggesting that we need to modify expectations from the current state of expectations by developing the responsible citizen-patient model to replace a strict consumerist model. That model would engender a set of responsibilities that encourage regaining and maintaining of a state of maximum health that accompanies the right to healthcare. This concept requires further development but some of the groundwork has begun with articulation of techniques that measure patient activation.[44] Clearly if we are serious about reducing healthcare costs, we must find a humane way to have patients be accountable for their part in healthcare while keeping healthcare professionals accountable and engaged in the face of the Other. Wikler and Brock raise the issue of individual responsibility for health in their consideration of population-level bioethics, but question whether it is a matter of social injustice or personal responsibility.[45] Clearly a population perspective challenges the consumerist view of healthcare. The American dilemma in healthcare requires envisioning a new model of healthcare responsibilities and accountabilities while preserving access to healthcare for the less engaged patient. It is a change that requires a delicate balance of rights and responsibilities and an effort to preserve the humaneness of clinical practice. Both parties, the caregiver and the cared-for need to make a serious effort to make the relationship work. But as Bauman notes the precariousness of social existence and business connections inspires a desire for immediate consumption and gratification to the detriment of lasting human bonds that need the nurturing by both parties.[46] Of course the postmodern clinical encounter has several other parties including insurers, healthcare delivery systems, regulatory bureaucracies, and patient advocacy groups. The clinical dyad is subsumed in the complex postmodern healthcare nexus.

THE NOT-SO-PROFITABLE HEALTHCARE ORGANIZATION

The for-profit healthcare industry has contributed to healthcare costs and expenditures. The decision to make healthcare a for-profit industry was a fateful one. While it is unrealistic to think that the healthcare industry can be turned into an entirely not-for-profit one, it may be reasonable to implement measures that reduce the single-minded pursuit of profits. In fact, the Patient Protection and Affordable Care Act limits the profits and administration costs to 20 percent of the premium pool.[47]

Business ethicist Thomas O'Brien notes that the aggrandizing forces in corporations are too myopically focused on profit, and that business leadership needs to change in the direction of recognizing the common good.[48] Bauman notes that, "In the universe of technology, the moral self with its negligence of rational calculation, disdain of practical uses, and indifference to pleasure, feels and is an unwelcome alien,"[49] Our society needs to welcome the "alien" moral self to the table, so to speak, and ask that moral self back into our midst amid corporate enterprises and contend more with the ethical aspects of the organization of healthcare delivery. To begin with, legislation could require that every healthcare organization have a significant plurality of board members from the healthcare provider side (physician and nurse), patient representatives and a bioethicist or two to provide a voice for ethical practice in healthcare delivery. Board members of healthcare organizations should also require a minimum number that are women because 50.7 percent of Americans are female, and because they are *somewhat* more likely to be person-centered than profit-centered. O'Brien notes that the distorted prioritization of profit maximization needs a corrective of concern for the common good.[50] Postmodern thought needs to reach out for new methods of deconstructing the power accretion and concentration by the mega-corporations of the twenty-first century in order to provide mechanisms to humanize them and counterbalance their obsessive pursuit of profit over all other social goods. Perhaps requiring that hospital and healthcare system either their CEOs or COOs be physicians or nurses instead of having MBAs rule the healthcare industry with a singular business focus. Goodall notes that sixteen out of twenty-one CEOs of the top ranked hospitals by *US News and World Report* are physicians.[51] Perhaps having physicians in leadership roles may improve quality of care, if not make them more ethically sensitive. A relaxation of the singular focus on the return on investment may improve the ethos and/or quality of care. Postmodern thinkers have unfinished tasks to further deconstruct the power aggrandizement of healthcare corporations and re-humanize the healthcare industry on postmodern terms. The healthcare social fabric needs renewal.

MINDFUL MEDICAL PRACTICE AND CARING FOR THE OTHER

From Levinas and Bauman, one can discern an outline of the immanent ethic of responsibility for the Other. As previously noted, some degree of reciprocity is needed to nurture the natural moral intuitions regarding altruism and caring. There is surely more focus on the character and development of the medical professional but some degree of reciprocity needs the human face of caring. Good appropriately critiques Foucault for ignoring the importance of the dialogical nature of discourse and the importance of lived experience of disease and healthcare.[52] Physicians similarly can be indifferent to the life experiences of their patients and patients generally reciprocate that indifference. Can mindfulness training of physicians reverse this trend?

To engage a significant percentage of postmodern professionals in practicing an ethos of caring may require changes in medical education. Already a growing number of medical schools are teaching its students mindfulness training as an elective.[53] Mindfulness training increases self-awareness, the first component of emotional intelligence.[54] Self-awareness and self-control, awareness of others' feelings and how one influences those feelings are crucial to being an effective postmodern healthcare provider. Here too balance should be sought between a focus on self-understanding and self-control and understanding others.

More than three decades ago, Kabat-Zinn started a movement that has brought mindfulness training to patients with chronic medical and psychological conditions.[55] Ludwig and Kabat-Zinn see mindfulness training as an antidote to the "continuous partial attention" of our rapid sequencing computerized world.[56] Shapiro et al. found that mindfulness training increased empathy and decreased stress levels in medical students as compared to controls.[57] It would appear that it can increase the degree to which students are aware of the Other. It is very encouraging that an increasing number of medical schools including those at the University of Pennsylvania, University of Rochester, and Drexel University are offering mindfulness training. Previously an ethos of affective distancing and emotional detachment was favored in medical schools but that may be changing in favor of more empathic engagement.[58] Hojat et al., in a study of declining empathy in the third year of medical school when students begin regularly working with patients, observed that such factors as overly-demanding patients and lack of appreciation by patients contributed to the decline.[59] The need for reflexivity and mutuality is clearly needed in the clinical encounter. Patients too need to have some awareness of the Other as healthcare provider for this model of interaction to flourish. The consumerist ethos is antithetical to a culture of collaboration. A remarkable change in how media communicate about healthcare providers needs the involvement of physician and nursing organizations to explain their challenges and difficulties to the patient population.

Mindfulness can help prevent burnout as well as enhance empathy in clinicians. Krasner, Epstein, et al. have demonstrated in practicing primary care physicians, a group somewhat disposed to burnout for a variety of a factors, that mindfulness training along with appreciative inquiry and other approaches can increase empathy while reducing burnout.[60] What remains to be seen is whether such techniques also work in groups of physicians not self-selected for participation in such efforts. An approach to mindfulness appears to be a promising approach for expanding the Levinasian ideal in medical practice.

APPRECIATIVE INQUIRY IN THE MEDICAL CENTER: OSUMC

A group of academic physician leaders at the Ohio State University Medical Center were engaged in a comprehensive effort to enhance medical professionalism in an effort they have termed, "Turning Around the Titanic: Implemented a Culture of Professionalism at a Large Academic Medical Center."[61]

This is an apt metaphor for attempting to change the academic medical industrial complex as it drifts towards a sort of moral "iceberg." Led by the Interim Dean of the Ohio State College of Medicine, Catherine R. Lucey, MD and Cynthia Ledford, MD, Chair of the Professionalism Council, this was a multi-pronged approach that recognized the need to change the professionalism paradigm from one based on virtue to one based on a sustainable skills approach.[62] These skills include self awareness, self-control, diplomacy, and resilience. The concept is extended to include medical students, resident physicians as well as attending physicians to develop and apply these skills in clinical situations. These skills should be brought to bear when having difficult discussions with patients and families about serious prognoses, disclosing medical errors, when colleagues and employees are shirking responsibilities or demonstrating disruptive behavior, or when discussing poor performance with trainees by making use of techniques of appreciative inquiry, best practices, executive coaching, appreciative performance improvement feedback and other postmodern management techniques. It was a very ambitious, comprehensive effort and the Titanic does not turn easily.

While I am inclined to describe this approach as communitarian and pragmatic, it could also be depicted as the application of postmodern management techniques. Leadership development, appreciative inquiry, and techniques of executive coaching have a stronger foundation in the business world today than in healthcare delivery. I am not surprised that female leaders were strongly involved in this effort although many men were as well. Healthcare delivery can benefit from such management techniques as well as having leaders embrace the foundational values of medical practice. The sphere of medicine can add something not usually found in business, however: a tradition of interest, concern and dedication for the Other, the patient. If a balance of normativity to performativity can be initiated in the academic medical center, then it can also be accomplished in other healthcare organizations. This may be a too optimistic view of the possible. If our epistemes are our destiny and we become more mindful of the content of our current epistemes, we may be able to improve the moral milieu. Kovacs has observed that in our pluralistic culture, only a "soft form of ethical expertise" is imaginable.[63] What is possible then is a type of *pros hen* ethical pluralism that Ess notes "requires shared but not always identical points of ethical agreement and acknowledges that there are multiple agents with varying judgments."[64] What develops is not exactly moral consensus but is a thinner type of agreement. A society needs some agreement on its core values.

Bauman reminds us that, "Morality which we inherited from pre-modern times is a morality of proximity, and as so such inadequate in a society in which all important action is an action at a distance."[65] Capturing some closeness in the cyber age is a necessary challenge.

THE FUTURE OF POSTMODERN MEDICAL CARE

Communitarianism did not succeed because of the atomistic nature of post-modern life. Although we dwell in a sphere of moral relativism, it does not need to result in moral nihilism. The moral intuitions that arise within the human can be further studied and communicated; epistemes can be developed to better reflect the social reality of institutions, laws, social mores and related phenomena. Bauman has noted that the *raison d'etre* of the development of ethics is social ordering.[66] It is debatable how well our current ethos has accomplished this. Every social ordering has elements of injustice and arbitrariness, as Foucault helped us to understand. However, from the perspective of providing medical care in the twenty-first century, we can discern an outline of the project to preserve the ethos of medical professionalism in an environment sometimes hostile to ethical considerations and medical professionals alike. The myth of physician superiority has been vanquished decisively but new myths of superiority of computerized systems have risen to take its place. Computerization also challenges the healthcare environment to focus on great volumes of data (the Silicon Cage) which could further dehumanize medical practice. Great vigilance will be needed to avoid that from happening. Will the postmodern medical bureaucracies be constrictive of creativity and humaneness? Or can they find a way, after Deleuze and Guattari, to be rhizomatic in their nature, achieving a balance between regulation, and creative and dynamic human consciousness? I believe that some of the better healthcare organizations are already trying to reach this balance between an orderly bureaucracy and a space for human creativity, yet many have not taken this approach.

The Taoist concept of *wu wei* denotes effortless doing or creative quietude, a creating of a space of opportunity for the expression of the natural human essence.[67] Mindfulness training helps expands this space of quiet engagement, but can large technocratic bureaucracies accommodate this space temporally as well as conceptually? An approach that leaves room for humane expression of caring can complement in important ways the strong focus on the massive accumulation of data. It can also be a moderating influence on the development of the next fundamental changes in delivering medical care as well as training clinicians.

Humankind has a need to discover, as best it can, the preconditions for inter-subjective relations that are authentic, caring, and enduring so that the face of the Other shines in our own. Levinas cautions that one cannot countenance the face of the Other without the proper language that embraces "affective intentionality."[68] I submit we will not find that affective intentionality in the various medical computer systems, regimented bureaucracy, or the corporate practice of medicine.

For medical care to flourish in postmodern times, patients as well as providers need to be educated and responsible for their parts, the profit motive needs to take a less prominent role, and the robustness of the human dialogue that is at the center of the clinical encounter needs to be nourished and treated with respect and dignity. With the leveling of the medical hierarchy under the influence of postmodernism, it is fair to ask what constitutes the moral agency or responsibility of the patient and healthcare organizations. I propose the development of the "not-so-profitable healthcare organization" as one that embraces an ethical value in addition to profitability. Otherwise the commodification of medical practice endangers the moral engagement in clinical care. As Borgmann noted, "commodification creates a detachment of a good or service from its context of engagement with a place, time, and a community."[69] We have ceased to a have a community of healers when commodification of healthcare is completely computerized and clinical decisions are made top down. These circumstances have arrived rapidly as the healthcare industry implemented with certitude the Silicon Cage, slighting the humanistic aspects of medical practice.

Levinas has provided guidance in how to feel morally responsible for another person, and he suggests this is possible even in the absence of reciprocity. I am not sure that is true at all. It is not easy to possess the sensibility without something akin to gratitude. The heart of the ethical practice of medicine nevertheless requires that we attempt to do so. By challenging ourselves as well as the received wisdom of our time, a thorough investigation of the postmodern condition and postmodern thought can help advance this effort. We must heed Roy Porter's warning that medicine must redefine its limits and our expectations realistically with a greater understanding of the socio-cultural milieu that postmodern culture has created for healthcare as well as to better understand the role of its crucial stakeholders, patients, clinicians, and its myriad of related institutions.

NOTES

1. Bauman Z. *Postmodern Ethics*. Oxford UK: Blackwell 2000, p. 60.

2. Jencks C. *The postmodern agenda in The Postmodern Agenda*. London: Academic Books. 1992.

3. Porter R. *The Greatest Benefit to Mankind*. New York: Norton, 1998.

4. McCollough T. E. *The Moral Imagination and Public Life: Raising the Ethical Question*. Chatham N.J.: Chatham Books. 1992. P72.

5. Giroux H. *Stealing Innocence: Youth, Corporate Power, and the Politics of Culture:* New York Palgrave. 2000. P. 172.

6. Poses R. M. A cautionary tale: the dysfunction of American health care. *Eur J Int Med* 14(2):123–130, 2003.

7. Relman A. S. The new medical industrial complex. *N Engl J Med* 303(17):963–970, 1980.

8. Brawley O. W., Goldberg P. *How We Do Harm: A Doctor Breaks Ranks about Being Sick in America*. New York: St. Martins Press 2012.

9. Norris T. Hannah Arendt & Jean Baudrillard: Pedagogy in the Consumer Society. *Studies in Philosophy and Education* 25:457–77, 2006.

10. Baudrillard J. The consumer society in *Jean Baudrillard Selected Writings*, M. Poster (ed). Stanford Univ Press 2001, p. 41.

11. Goold S. D., Neblo M. A., S. Y. H. Kim, et al. What is Good Public Deliberation? *Hastings Ctr Rep* 42(2):24–26, 2012.

12. Pear R. US Backs Oregon Healthcare Plan for the Poor New York Times. March 23, 1003. http://www.nytimes.com/1993/03/20/us/us-backs-oregon-s-health-plan-for-covering-all-poor-people.html. Accessed December 15, 2012.

13. Steinberg R. J., edit. *Wisdom:Its Nature, Origins, and Development*. New York: Cambridge Univ. Press 2000.

14. Hall S. S. *Wisdom: From Philosophy to Neuroscience*. New York: Vintage 2010. P247.

15. J.-K. Choi, S. Bowles. The co evolution of parochial altruism and war. *Science* 318: 636–640, 2007.

16. De Dreu C. K. W., Greer L. L., et al. The Neuropeptide Oxytocin Regulates Parochial Altruism in Intergroup Conflict Among Humans. *Science* 328:1408–1411, 2010.

17. Zygmunt B. *Postmodern Ethics*. Blackwell, Oxford 1993, p14.

18. Habermas J. *Habermas and Modernity*. Edit. Bernstein R. J. MIT Press 1984, p. 86.

19. Borgmann 1984, 41.

20. Fallman D. A different way of seeing: Albert Borgmann's philosophy of technology and human-computer interaction. *AI & Soc* 25:53–60, 2010.

21. CMS HER incentive programs https://www.cms.gov/Regulations-and-Guidance/Legislation/EHRIncentivePrograms/Downloads/Stage2Overview_Tipsheet.pdf Accessed December 2012.

22. The Leapfrog Group. http://www.leapfroggroup.org/news/leapfrog_news/4779269 Accessed Dec 16, 2012.

23. Wychgrod E. *Emmanuel Levinas: The Problem of Ethics Metaphysicis*. New York: Fordham Univ Press 200. Chapter 1. Early Themes.

24. Clifton-Soderstrom M. Levinas and the Patient as Other: The Ethical Foundation of Medicine. *J Med Phil* 28(4): 447–460, 2010.

25. McCullough M. C. E., Kimeldorf M. B., Cohen A. D. An Adaptation for Altruism? Current Directions in Psychological Science, 17, 281–284, 2008.

26. Azetsop J., Rennie S. Principlism, medical individualism, and health promotion in resource-poor countries: can autonomy-based bioethics promote social justice and population health? *Philosophy, Ethics, and Humanities in Medicine* 5:1–10, 2010.

27. Ibid. p. 4.

28. Nash D. B., Reifsnyder J., Fabius R., Pracilio V. P. Population Health: Creating a Culture of Wellness. *Sudbury MA Jones and Bartlett Learning* 2011.

29. Persad G., Wertheimer A., Emanuel E. J. Principles for allocation of scarce medical interventions. *Lancet* 273:423–31, 2009.

30. Elpern E. H., Covert B., Kleinpell R. Moral Distress of Staff Nurses in a Medical Intensive Care Unit. *Am J Crit Care* 14(6):523–530, 2005.

31. Zuzelo P. R. Exploring the Moral Distress of Registered Nurses. *Nursing Ethics.* 14(3):344–59, 2007.

32. Mannison R., Small N. Postmodern Health Economics. *Health Care Analysis* 7: 255–272, 1999.

33. Wilk R. Consuming Morality. *J Consumer Culture* 1:245–260, 2001.

34. Eiser A. R. & Weiss M. The Underachieving Advance Directive: Recommendations for Increasing Advance Directives Completion. *Am J Bioeth.* 1(4): W10, 2001.

35. Foucault M. *The Order of Things*. New York: Pantheon 1970.

36. Adler P., Borys B. Two types of bureaucracy: enabling and coercive. *Administr, Sci Quart* 61–89, 1996.

37. Gewirtz S. Ethical Reflexivity in policy analysis: what is it and why do we need it? *Praxis Educativa, Ponta Grassa* 2(1):7–12, 2007.

38. Hibbard J. H., Stockard J., Mahoney E. R., et al. Development of Patient Activation Measure (PAM): conceptualizing and measuring activation in patients and consumers. *Health Ser Res* 39:1005–1026, 2004.

39. Becker E. R., Robbin D. W. Translating Primary Care Practice Climate into Patient Activation. *Med Care* 46(8):795–805, 2008.

40. Borgmann A. *Holding On to Reality: The Nature of Information at the Turn of the Millennium.* Univ Chicago Press 1999, p. 221.

41. Howard J. S. Subjectivity and Space: Deleuze and Guattari's BwO in the New World Order. In *Deleuze and Guattari: New Mappings in Politics, Philosophy, and Culture.* Kaufman E., Heller J. K. Univ Minnesota Press 1998.

42. Wicks P, Vaughan TE, Massagli MP, Heywood J. Accelerated clinical discovery using self-reported patient data collected online and a patient-matching algorithm 1 Nature BiotechnologyVolume:29:Pages 411–414, 2011 Year published:DOI:

43. Detsky A. S. What Patient Really Want from Health Care. *JAMA* 306(22): 2500–01, 2011.

44. Hibbard J. H., Stockard J., E. R. Mahoney, and M. Tusler. Development of the Patient Activation Measure (PAM): Conceptualizing and Measuring Activation in Patients and Consumers. *Health Services Research* 39 (4): 1005–26, 2004.

45. Wikler D., Brock D. W. Population-Level Bioethics: Mapping a New Agenda. In *Ethics, prevention, and public health,* Dawson A. & Verweij M., p. 78. New York: Oxford University Press, 2007.

46. Bauman Z. *Liquid Modernity* Cambridge UK: Polity 2000, p. 164

47. http://www.dpc.senate.gov/healthreformbill/healthbill49.pdf Accessed June 15, 2013.

48. O'Brien T. Reconsidering the Common Good in the Business Context. *J Business Ethics.* 85:25–37, 2009.

49. Bauman. *Postmodern Ethics,* p. 198.

50. O'Brien. Ibid. p. 35.

51. . Goodall E. Physicians-Leaders and Hospital Performance: Is there an association? *AZA DP* 5830 http://www.amandagoodall.com/HospitalCEOsAssociationSSMMarch2011.pdf. Accessed July 6, 2011.

52. Good B. J. *Medicine, Rationality and Experience. An anthropological perspective.* Cambridge University Press 1994, p. 69.

53. O'Reilly K. B. Using mindfulness to sooth physician distress. *AMA News* Jan 7, 2013. http://www.amednews.com/article/20130107/profession/130109974/4/.

54. Goleman D. *Emotional Intelligence.* New York: Bantam. 2005.

55. Kabat-Zinn J. An outpatient program in behavioral medicine for chronic pain patients' base on the practice of mindfulness meditation. *Gen Hosp Psychiatry* 4(2): 33–47, 1982.

56. Ludwig D. Kabat-Zinn J. Mindfulness in Medicine. *JAMA* 300(11): 1350–1352, 2008.

57. Shapiro S. L., Schwartz G. E., Bonner G. Effects of mindfulness-based stress reduction on medical and pre-medical students. *J Behav. Med* 21(6): 581–599, 1998.

58. Halpern F. *From Detached Concern to Empathy: Humanizing Medical Practice.* NY: Oxford Univ Press, 2001.

59. Hojat M. *Empathy in Patient Care: Antecedents, Development, Measurement, and Outcomes.* New York, NY: Springer; 2007

60. Krassner R. M., Epstein R. M. Association of an educational program in mindful communication with burnout, empathy, and attitudes among primary care physicians. *JAMA* 302(12): 1284–93, 2009.

61. Lucey C. http://medicine.osu.edu/faculty/gov/professionalism/pages/index.aspx Accessed June 11, 2011.

62. Ledford C., Lucey C. http://medicine.osu.edu/faculty/gov/professionalism/pages/index. aspx Accessed Feb 2012.

63. Kovacs J. The transformation of (bio)ethics expertise in the world of ethical pluralism. *J Med Ethics* 36:767–770, 2010.

64. Ess C. Ethical pluralism and global information ethics. *Ethics & Information Tech.* 8:215–226, 2006.

65. Bauman Z. *Postmodern Ethics.* Oxford UK: Blackwell. 1993. P. 217.

66. Bauman. *Social Cohesion: Does Ethics Have a Chance in a World of Consumers?* Cambridge Mass, Harvard U Press 2008, p.

67. Ames R. T. "Wu-wei in 'The Art of Rulership' Chapter of Huai Nan Tzu." *Philosophy East and West* 31, no. 2 (April 1981): 196.

68. Wyschogrod E. *Emanuel Levinas: The Problem of Ethical Metaphysics.* New York: Fordham Univ Press. 2000, p. 231.

69. Borgmann A. The Here and Now: Theory, Technology, and Actuality. *Philo. Technol* 24:5–17, 2011.

Epilogue

Ethos of Medicine in Postmodern America

"Humility is a quality that demands careful titration, a delicate (and often shifting) balance between personal agency, social deference, the inner strength of self-awareness, and a good-humored grace in acknowledging human limitations." —Stephan S. Hall [1]

"The countermovement against impersonal rationality allows us not to forget that it is we who are seeing this society and world; it is not seeing itself through us." —Jeffery Alexander [2]

Looking back on my suggested recommendations in the last few chapters, I must acknowledge they are not strictly postmodern in nature because they contain some positivistic claims. While attempting to remain cognizant of the limitations of postmodernist thought, I am suggesting it is worthwhile to attempt to address the current systemic flaws that have developed in our overly commercialized healthcare delivery system. I am advocating for a *post-postmodern ethos* that offers a renewed consciousness of the Other through the implementation of both some very old techniques (mindfulness meditation) as well as some newer techniques for team building using advances in the neurosciences, postmodern management, and applied psychology.

As a physician, I cannot limit my efforts solely to critiquing the current state of medical affairs. I am too concerned about it and find a compelling need to attempt to improve the health of healthcare today. The problems with healthcare are hardly confined to the United States, being experienced in such diverse countries as the United Kingdom, China, Slovenia, and Japan.

Postmodern influences know no bounds as globalism, computerization, and consumerism penetrate the ethos far and wide. Some problematic features of healthcare delivery are unique to each country and jurisdiction, each community and its practitioners, healthcare and insurance executives, their policies, consumer features, and political environments. Some problems seem to be common to many different cultures, social circumstances, and economic settings, suggesting some overarching patterns and that even positivist claims are possible regarding healthcare delivery challenges. The United States, however, has a large lead over other countries in its degree of excessive healthcare consumption and expenditures. This matter has captured national attention and generated considerable political controversy. There are no easy solutions, and the healthcare debate deserves to have more sobriety and recognition of the limits of healthcare as well as its noteworthy accomplishments. The healthcare philosophy of maximizing human autonomy with its resultant permissiveness of unhealthy lifestyles with rescue by highly technical interventions late in the course of disease, activating an army of high tech, high cost interventionists is not economically viable in the long run. We need an ethos of healthy living and not merely of exponential increase in healthcare delivery.

Attempting to balance the strong forces of the expanding healthcare bureaucracies with the humanistic aspects of medical care is clearly an important project but how to do so is not yet clearly delineated. The challenge to create a balance will certainly not be solved by my suggestions alone. Hopefully I have pointed to the general direction where solutions may lie, and others may more clearly illuminate a path to more effective policies that preserve the humane aspects of the clinical encounter and the professional nature of medical practice. Postmodern thought can help us understand what has happened to the social fabric of healthcare delivery but cannot readily provide solutions except in the broadest outline. A pragmatic utilitarian approach may be needed but it must be one that has a realistic comprehension of human psychology, human limitations, and human capabilities.

I readily admit that I believe in the importance and the benefit of thorough and precise data analysis in healthcare quality improvement. Advances through such an approach have already yielded significant improvements. Yet at the same time I recognize the limits of quantitative data and how they easily can be misused and misinterpreted if confounding factors are not taken into consideration. As I discussed in several previous chapters, the risks are considerable in diminishing the role of the important unquantifiable, experiential, communicative, intuitive and interpersonal aspects of high quality medical care. Balancing between data collection and structured order sets on the one hand, and the cultivation of a human face in healthcare on the other is a nuanced, delicate task that must avoid broad strokes and archaic generalizations. The effort to preserve a humane professional identity for medical practitioners is essential to maintaining a worthwhile and respectful ethos of medical practice in the 21st century. Impersonal bureaucratic rationality will never suffice to comfort the sick, ease their suffering, and heal their wounded spirits. The computer, the corporation, and the consumerist model will not accomplish that. We still need men and women to face the suffering of the sick and patiently, personally provide that comforting and healing in an inter-subjective fashion with compassion, expertise, knowledge, humility, and respect. We cannot permit the Silicon Cage to envelop medical practice and vanquish the human spirit from the clinical encounter. We need to develop new insights and techniques through advances in neurosciences, neuroethics, and applied psychology. Ultimately we need to confront the moral relativism and fluidity of our era and attempt to forge a counter-development that improves and strengthens the moral tone of post-postmodern society.

NOTES

1. Hall Stephen S. *Wisdom: From Philosophy to Neuroscience*. Vintage: New York, 2011. P.138.
2. Alexander J. The Postpositivist Epistemological Dilemma in *Postmodernism & Social Theory*. Edit. Seidman S., Wagner D. G. Oxford: Blackwell 1992 p.329.

Selected Bibliography

Armstrong, D. Bodies of Knowledge/knowledge of bodies. In *Reassessing Foucault*, C. Jones, R. Porter (eds.). London: Routledge 1994.

Bell, D. *The Cultural Contradictions of Capitalism* New York: Basic Books, 1976.

Baudrillard, Jean. *Simulacra and Simulation*. Transl. Glaser S. F. Ann Arbor: U Mich Press, 1994.

Bauman, Zygmunt. *Globalization: The Consequences*. Cambridge UK: Polity Press 1998.

———. Collateral casualties of consumerism. *J. Consumer Culture* 25-56, 2007.

———. *Postmodernist Ethics*. Oxford: Blackwell, 1999.

———. *Liquid Modernity*. Cambridge, UK: Polity 2000.

———. *Does Ethics Have a Chance in a World of Consumers?* Cambridge, MA: Harvard U Press, 2008.

Borgmann, Albert. Holding on to reality. *The Nature of information at the Turn of the Millennium*. Chicago: Univ Chicago Press. 1999.

———. The Here and Now: Theory, Technology, and Actuality. *Philo. Technol* 24:5-17, 2011.

Clifton-Soderstrom, M. Levinas and the Patient as Other: The Ethical Foundation of Medicine *J Med Phil* 28(4): 447-460, 2003.

Dean, J. The Networked Empire. In *Empire's New Clothes: Reading Hardt and Negri*. Eds., Passavant P. A., Dean J. New York: Routledge. 2004.

Ellul, Jacques. *The Technological Society*. New York: Knopf. 1964.

Foucault, Michel. *The History of Sexuality vol1 An Introduction*. Trans R. Hurley. London: Penguin. 1980.

———. *Power/Knowledge: Selected Writings* 1972-1977. Ed. Gordon C. New York: Pantheon, 1980.

———. *The Birth of the Clinic: An Archeology of Medical Perception*. New York: Vintage 1973.

———. *The Archeology of Knowledge and the Discourse of Language*. Trans. A. M. Sheridan Smith. New York: Pantheon, 1972.

———. *Discipline and Punish: The Birth of the Prison*. Gallimard 1975.

Deleuze, Giles. *Foucault*. Transl. Sean Hand. Minneapolis: University of Minnesota Press, 1988.

———. *Capitalism and Schizophrenia*. Minneapolis: Univ Minnesota, 1987.

Deleuze, Giles and Guattari F. *A Thousand Plateaus*. Transl. Massoni B. Minneapolis: University of Minnesota Press, 1987.

Grant, I. H. Postmodernism and Science and Technology. In *Postmodernism*. Ed. Stuart Sim. Oxford and New York: Routledge, 2001 .

Giddens, A. Living in a Post-traditional society. In *Reflexive Modernization*. Eds. U. Beck, A. Giddens, S Lash. Cambridge: Polity Press, 1994.

Godzich, W. Afterword, *The Postmodern Explained*. J-F Lyotard. Univ Minnesota. 1992.

Jameson, F. *Postmodernism, or the Cultural Logic of Late Capitalism*. Durham NC: Duke Univ Press, 1991.

Holland, E. W. From Schizophrenia to Social Control. In Deleuze and Guattari, *New Mappings in Politics, Philosophy, and Culture*. University of Minnesota, 1998.

Hoogenboom, Marcel and Ossewaarde, Ringo. From Iron Cage to Pigeon House: The Birth of Reflexive Authority. *Organization Studies* 26(4): 601-619, 2005.

Howard, J. S. Deleuze and Guattari's *Born in the New World Order*. In *DeLeuze and Guattari: New Mappings in Politics, Philosophy, and Culture*. Kaufman E., Heller K. J. U Minnesota Press, 1998.

Kelemen, M., Peltonen T. Ethics, morality, and the subject: the contribution of Zygmunt Bauman and Michel Foucault to a business ethics. *Scandavian J Management*. 17(2): 151-66, 2001.

Kaufman, E., Heller, K. J. Deleuze and Guattari, *New Mappings in Politics, Philosophy, and Culture*. Univ Minnesota Press, 1998.

Levinas, Emanuel. *Alterity and Transcendence*. Transl. M. B. Smith. Columbia University Press NY, 1999.

———. *Basic Philosophical Writings*. Ed. Peperzak A. T., Critchley S., Bernaasconi R. Indiana U Press, 1996.

———. *Totality and Infinity: An Essay on Exteriority*. Transl. Lingis A. Pittsburgh: Duquesne University Press, 1969.

Lyotard, Jean-Francois. *The Postmodern Condition: A Report on Knowledge*. Trans. Bennington G., Massumi B. University Minnesota Press,1984.

———. *The Differend: Phrases in Dispute*. Trans. G. Van Den Abbeele. Minneapolis: Univ Minn Press,1991.

———. Thiebaud J-L. *Just Gaming*. Trans. Godzich W. Minneapolis: Minnesota Univ Press, 1985.

———. *The Post Modern Explained*. Minneapolis: University of Minnesota Press, 1993.

Massaide, P. Possibly abusive, often benign, always necessary. On power and domination in medical practice. *Sociol Health Illness* 13:545-561, 1991.

Morris, David. *Illness and Culture in the Postmodern Age*. Berkeley: Univ. Calif Press, 1998.

Nuyen, A. T. Lyotard's postmodern ethics and information technology. *Ethics Inform Tech* 6:185-191, 2004.

Seidman, S. *Postmodern Social Theory as Narrative in Postmodernism & Social Theory*. Eds. Seidman S., Wagner D. G. Blackwell: Oxford, 1992, 47-81.

Sheridan, A. *Michel Foucault: The Will to Truth*. London: Tavistock, 1980.

Wyschogrod, E. *Emanuel Levinas: The Problem of Ethical Metaphysics*. New York: Fordham Univ Press, 2000.

OTHER PHILOSOPHICAL THOUGHT

Azetsop, J., Rennie, S. Principlism, medical individualism, and health promotion in resource-poor countries: can autonomy-based bioethics promote social justice and population health? *Ethics and Humanities* 5:1, 2010. http://www.peh-med.com/content/5/1/1 Accessed Feb 1, 2011.

Habermas, Jurgen. *The Theory of Communicative Action*. Trans. McCarthy, Thomas. Boston: Beacon Press, 1984.

McIntyre, Alysdair. *After Virtue: A Study in Moral Theory*. South Bend, IN: Notre Dame U Press, 1984.

Polanyi, Michael. *Personal Knowledge: Toward a Post-Critical Philosophy*. London: Routledge & Kegan Paul, 1958.

Reinders, H. The importance of tacit knowledge in practices of care. *J Intellect Disab Res* 54 (suppl 1): 28-37, 2010.

Toulmin, Stephen E. *Medical institutions and their moral constraints*, in *Integrity in Health-care Institutions*. E. Bulger, Reiser S. J. (eds.). Iowa City: University of Iowa Press, 1990.

Weber, Max. *The Theory of Social and Economic Organization*. Trans. by A. M. Henderson and Talcott Parsons. London: Collier Macmillan Publishers, 1947.

PROFESSIONALISM

Brody, H. *Hooked: Ethics, the Medical Profession and the Pharmaceutical Industry*. Lanham: Rowman & Littlefield, 2007.

Caronna, M. C. A., Shortell, S. M. From the doctor's workshop to the iron cage? Evolving modes of physician control in US health systems. *Soc Scien Med* 60:1311-1322, 2005.

Cruise, J. History of Medicine: The Metamorphosis of Scientific Medicine in the Ever-Present Past. *Am J Med Sci* 318(3): 171-184, 1999.

Freidson, E. *Professionalism: The Third Logic*. Chicago: Univ Chicago Press, 2001.

Fiscella K., Meldrum S., Franks P., et al. Patient Trust: Is it Related to Patient-Centered Behavior of Primary Care Physicians? *Medical Care* 42(11): 1049-1055, 2004.

Halpern, J. *From Detached Concern to Empathy: Humanizing Medical Practice*. NY: Oxford Univ Press, 2001.

Light, D., Levine, S. The Changing Character of the Medical Profession: A Theoretical Overview. Milbank Quarterly 66(suppl. 2):10–32, 1988.

Mallon, Bill. *Ernest Amory Codman: The End Result of a Life in Medicine* . Philadelphia: WB Saunders, 2000.

Maseide, P. The deep play of medicine: Discursive and collaborative processing of evidence in medical problem solving. *Communication Med* 3(1): 43-54, 2006.

Owens, Dorothy. *Hospitality to Strangers: Empathy and the Physician-Patient Relationship*. Atlanta: Scholars Press, 1999.

Poses, R. M. A cautionary tale: the dysfunction of American health care. *Eur J Int Med* 14:123-130, 2003.

Redman, B., Yarandi H. M., Merz J. F. Empirical developments in retraction. *J Med Ethics* 34:807-9, 2008.

Steen, R. G. Retractions in the medical literature: how many patient are put at risk by flawed research. *J Med Ethics* 10:1136, 37 : 113-117, 2011.

Shanafelt, T. D., Boone, S., Tan, L. et al. Burnout and satisfaction with work-life balance among US physicians relative to the US population. *Arch Intern Med* 172:1377-1385, 2012.

HEALTH SERVICE RESEARCH

Casalino, L. The unintended consequences of measuring quality on the quality of medical care. *NEJM* 341:1147-1150, 1999.

Chassin, M. R. Achieving and maintaining improved quality: lessons from New York State and cardiac surgery. *Health Aff*. 21(4)40–51, 2002.

Davidoff F., Batalden P., Stevens D., Ogrinic G., Mooney S. Publication guidelines for improvement studies in healthcare: evolution of the SQUIRE project. *Ann Intern Med* 149:670–676, 2008.

Eddy, D. M. Performance Measurement: Problems and Solutions. *Health Aff* 17(4): 7-26, 1998.

―――. Health Technology Assessment and Evidence-Based Medicine: What Are We Talking About? *Value In Health Aff* 12(Suppl2) S6–S7, 2009.

―――. Clinical Decision Making: From theory into practice-anatomy of a decision. *JAMA* 263(3):441-443, 1990.

―――. Performance Measurement: Problems and Solutions. *Health Affairs* 17(4): 7-25, 1998.

Groopman J., Hartzband P. Why Quality of Care is Dangerous. *Wall Street Journal* April 8, 2009.

Hartzband P., Groopman J. Untangling the Web-Patients, Doctors, and the Internet. *NEJM* 362(12): 1063-6, 2010.

Institute of Medicine. *Clinical practice guidelines we can trust.* Washington, DC: Academies Press, 2011,

Jennings B., Baily M. A., Bottrell M., Lynn J., eds. *Heath Care Quality Improvement: Ethical and RegulatoryIssues.* http://www.thehastingscenter.org/Publications/SpecialReports/Detail.aspx?id=1342.

Lexchin J., Light D. W. Commercial influence and the content of medical journals. *BMJ* 332:1444-1446, 2006.

Makary, M. *Unaccountable: What Hospitals Won't Tell You and How Transparency Can Revolutionize Health Care.* New York: Bloomsbury: 2012 and Newsweek September 24, 2012.

Norheim, O. F. *The role of formal outcome evaluations in health policy making: a normative approach.* In *Evidenced-based Practice in Medicine and Healthcare,* Meulen R. T., Biller-Andorno N., Lenk C., Lie R., eds. Berlin: Springer Verlag 2005.

Powell A. A., White K. M., Partin M. R., et al. Unintended consequences of implementing a national performance measurement system into local practice. *J Gen Int Med* 27(4): 405-12, 2011.

Raspe, H. *Clinical evaluative research: which patient benefit, how and when? A contribution to a European discussion.* In *Evidenced-based Practice in Medicine and Healthcare,* ch. 12. Meulen R. T., Biller-Andorno N., Lenk C., Lie R., eds. Berlin: Springer Verlag 2005.

Richardson E. T., Polyakova A. The illusion of scientific objectivity and the death of the investigator. *Eur J Clin Invest* 42:213-215, 2011.

Rutledge, R. An analysis of 25 Milliman & Robertson Guidelines for Surgery: Data driven versus Consensus Derived Clinical Practice Guidelines. *Annals Surgery* 228(4):579-587.

Tunis, S. R. Reflections on science, judgment, and value in evidence-based decision making: a conversation with David Eddy. *Health Affairs* 26(4): 500-515, 2007.

Thygeson M., Morrisey L., Ulstad V. Adaptive leadership and the practice of medicine: complexity-based approach to reframing the doctor-patient relationship. *J. Eval. Clin Practice* 16:1009-15, 2010.

Vos, Houtepen, and Horstma. Evidence based medicine and power shifts in health care systems. *Health Care Analysis* 10:319-328, 2002.

Woodhandler S., Himmelstein D. Why pay for performance may be incompatible with quality improvement. *BMJ* 345: 50-51, 2012.

BUSINESS ETHICS AND BIOETHICS

Barlett D. L., Steele J. B. *Critical Condition: How Health Care in America Became Big Business & Bad Medicine.* New York: Doubleday, 2004.

Eiser A. R., Goold S. D., Suchman A. L. Bioethics and Business Ethics in the Management of Healthcare. *J Gen Int Med* 14: S58-62, 1999.

.Frederick, W. C. *Values, Nature and Culture in the American Corporation.* New York: Oxford U Press, 1995.

Freeman, E. *Strategic Management: A Stakeholder Approach.* Cambridge Univ Press, 1984.

Robert, J. *Moral Mazes.* New York: Oxford University Press,1988.

Robinson, James C. *The Corporate Practice of Medicine.* Berkeley: Univ California,1999.

OTHER REFERENCES

Angel, Marcia. *The Truth about Drug Companies: How They Deceive Us and What to Do About It.* New York: Random House, 2004.

Bodenheimer, T. Uneasy Alliance-Clinical Investigators and the pharmaceutical industry. *N Engl J Med* 342:1539-1544, 2000.

Brody, Howard. *The Future of Bioethics*. Oxford: Oxford Univ Press, 2009.

Denzin N. K., Lincoln Y. S., Giardina M. D. Disciplining qualitative research. *Int J Qual Studies in Education* 19(6):769-782, 2006.

Kabat-Zinn J. An outpatient program in behavioral medicine for chronic pain patients' base on the practice of mindfulness meditation. *Gen Hosp Psychiatry* 4(2): 33-47, 1982.

Ludwig D., Kabat-Zinn J. Mindfulness in Medicine. *JAMA* 300(11):1350-1352, 2008.

Krasner M. S., Epstein R. M., Beckman H., et al. Associaton of an educational program in mindful communication without burnout, empathy, attitudes among primary care physicians. *JAMA* 302(12):1284-93, 2009.

Pho, Kevin. Commentary on Kevin MD. *How patient satisfaction can kill*. http://www.kevinmd.com/blog/2012/02/patient-satisfaction-kill.html. Accessed November, 2012.

Rosenberg, C. *The Care of Strangers: The Rise of America's Hospital System*. New York: Basic Books, 1987.

Wynia M., Boren D. Better Regulation of Industry-Sponsored Clinical Trials Is Long Overdue. *J Law, Med, Ethics* 37: 410-419, 2009.

Index